AYAHUASCA AWAKENING

The Truth Behind the Amazon Jungle's Sacred Plant Medicine

By

Naomi Harper

This content is provided with the sole purpose of providing relevant information on a specific topic for which every reasonable effort has been made to ensure that it is both accurate and reasonable. Nevertheless, by purchasing this content you consent to the fact that the author, as well as the publisher, are in no way experts on the topics contained herein, regardless of any claims as such that may be made within. As such, any suggestions or recommendations that are made within are done so purely for entertainment value. It is recommended that you always consult a professional prior to undertaking any of the advice or techniques discussed within.

This is a legally binding declaration that is considered both valid and fair by both the Committee of Publishers Association and the American Bar Association and should be considered as legally binding within the United States.

Furthermore, the information that can be found within the pages described forthwith shall be considered both accurate and truthful when it comes to the recounting of facts. As such, any use, correct or incorrect, of the provided information will render the Publisher free of responsibility as to the actions taken outside of their direct purview. Regardless, there are zero scenarios where the original author or the Publisher can be deemed liable in any fashion for any damages or hardships that may result from any of the information discussed herein.

Additionally, the information in the following pages is intended only for informational purposes and should thus be thought of as universal. As befitting its nature, it is presented without assurance regarding its prolonged validity or interim quality. Trademarks that are mentioned are done without written consent and can in no way be considered an endorsement from the trademark holder.

This book is intended for informational purposes only. People wishing to drink Ayahuasca should consult their medical doctors before engaging with this medicine. The use, possession, and trafficking of Ayahuasca is illegal in many countries, and the author does not condone the breaking of the laws of any country.

TABLE OF CONTENTS

Introduction 1

Chapter 1 *What Is Ayahuasca?* 3

The History of Ayahuasca 3

The Growing Popularity of Aya 5

Chapter 2 *The Science Of Ayahuasca* 7

The Components of Ayahuasca 7

How Ayahuasca Affects the Brain 7

How the Shamans Work with the Ayahuasca Vine 8

The Science of Ayahuasca Tea 10

How Ayahuasca Tea Affects the Brain 11

The Spiritual Effect of Ayahuasca Tea 13

How Admixtures Affect the Tea 14

Warnings about Admixtures 16

The Male Counterpart 17

Chapter 3 *Ayahuasca Ceremonies* 19

Shaman or a Charlton? 19

How Much Does a Ceremony Cost 22

The Breakdown of the Ceremony 23

Traditional Shaman Ceremony 24

Therapeutic Ceremony 28

Religious Ceremonies 29

Tips to Assist During the Ceremony 29

What Experiences to Expect 33

The Sexual Aspect 42

Redefining Your Ego as You Know It 44

The Process of Dissolution & Death of the Ego 46

Chapter 4 *Ayahuasca's Healing Powers* 49

The General Benefits.. 50
Post-Traumatic Stress Disorder 53
Depression and Anxiety 54
Cancer 54
Addictions 54
Mental Health Disorders 55
Overall Health Benefits 55
Health Risks with Ayahuasca Tea & Pharmaceutical Medicine 57
Spiritual Benefits 58
Chapter 5 *How To Get The Most Out Of Your Journey With Ayahuasca* 61
Choose Your Setting 61
Find Peace 62
Set a Heightened Awareness Intention 62
The Emotional Rollercoaster 63
Watch What You Consume 64
Prepare Yourself Mentally for the Journey 65
Choosing the Best Shaman for You 66
Use your Intuition 67
Inner Work Homework 67
Trust & Respect 69
Helpful Restrictions 69
Be Aware of Cultural Differences 69
Get Comfortable 70
Integration Success 70
Coming Back to the Real World 71
Your Health is Important 71
Conclusion 75
Description 76

INTRODUCTION

Congratulations on purchasing your copy of Ayahuasca Awakening: The Truth Behind the Amazon Jungle's Sacred Plant Medicine.

For the last four decades, there has been an explosion of interest in ayahuasca tea as it has created a windstorm of multiple layers of transformation mentally, physically and spiritually for countless people around the world. Some of the participants are simply backpackers who are looking for a story to tell when they get back from their travels. Some are people who specifically take a trip to South America to seek a Shaman or retreat center to partake in therapeutic sessions for medical reasons. Others have the absolute need for spiritual transcendence and are looking for clarity on the reason why they are here. They seek spiritual guidance from their infinite knowledge contained within their conscious and wish to travel to other indescribable astral dimensions to obtain this clarity of understanding of the world.

This is the perfect book for the beginner to know what to expect during their first ayahuasca experience. It is important to know that no matter how much knowledge that you gain about Aya, you will find that you will have a much deeper understanding once you have the opportunity to try the brew journey for yourself. The path to Mother Ayahuasca is personal to each person and can only be defined on an individual level.

You will learn about the history of ayahuasca tea as well as the transformations that have occurred in the ayahuasca tourism industry since the massive spread of information about this transformative brew. The science and how the ayahuasca tea affects the mechanism of your brain which then bleed over into the spiritual aspects of yourself will also be explained.

There is a complete overview of the different types of ceremonies that you can attend while focusing on a trip to the Amazon Rainforest. Preparation tips as well as insights into personal and scientific accounts are included to show the validity of the application of the ancient medicine which has been healing people all over the world successfully.

There is an overview of the medical concerns as well as ways to ensure that you take as much as possible away with you after the ceremony. The integration period is crucial to apply what you have learned from Madre Aya in a deep and meaningful way. Ego Death as well as the transformation of your ego during this process is given as a guide in this comprehensive completion of everything that you need to know.

There are plenty of books on Ayahuasca, and thanks again for choosing this one! Every effort was made to ensure that it is full of as much useful information as possible.

CHAPTER 1

What Is Ayahuasca?

The History of Ayahuasca

There are a multitude of indigenous communities in South America that use the vine of ayahuasca as a healing measure for ailments as well as a facilitator to conduct treatments and healings. Since there are no written records as to when this practice started, it is hard to pinpoint exactly how long ayahuasca has been used by Shamans as a healing medicine. However, there are oral records of one indigenous community's ayahuasca brew recipe being created 5,000 years ago.

Spanish and Portuguese missionaries came over to South America during the 16th century and came in contact with the ayahuasca using indigenous South Americans. In their closed minded ideal, they believed that the healing work of the plant was the devil's work and sparked controversy on its use between their different cultures and belief systems. They never inquired about the healing properties of ayahuasca and, as such, ayahuasca was virtually unknown outside of the Amazon region until the 20th century.

It was in 1908 that scientists in the west recognized the existence of ayahuasca and the mystical effects it had. This can be accredited to Richard Spruce, a British botanist, who came to South America to classify the tea's ingredients. He also wrote about the medicines purging effects as well as the significance of this master plant concoction to the culture of the Amazonian people.

Purging is a religious and cultural belief in which the purpose is to release all the negativity that has been blocking energy from correctly flowing through your subtle energy body as well as your physical body. This is done through several methods, but the most common are diarrhea and vomiting. Ayahuasca was also specifically to rid the body of parasites and worms. The Shamans believe the negative energies are the reason for illness and disease and should be a welcome aspect rather than a revolting ideal.

Interest in the spiritual and healing properties of ayahuasca was yet again peaked in the 1960s when the books were written by Richard Evans Schultes and brothers Dennis & Terance McKenna. These books were titled *The Yage Letters* and *True Hallucinations*, respectively. They recounted their personal experiences they had while using the ayahuasca brew in the Amazon. Even with the hippie and psychedelic movement going on at the time, the interest in this healing master plant had not spread worldwide as you still needed to take a trip to the Amazon rainforest at the time.

Master Plants are the most powerful teachers in the natural world. They are able to communicate with those who have had a close relationship with them over a long duration of time. They are able to build a respectful, trusting relationship with the plant and the spirit of the plant while being directed to the uses of that plant and perhaps others that will aid in the overall goal. The Shamans refer to these plants as *doctores* which is the Spanish name for *doctor* because the plants very much act the part.

The account from Schultes inspired journalist William S. Burroughs to go to the Amazon in search of a treatment or even a cure for opiate addictions. He was accompanied by psychiatrist Claudio Narajo by making the trip up the Amazon River in a canoe during the early 1970s. Narajo scientifically studied ayahuasca with the South American Indians and then later published *The Healing Journey* which included his findings of the active alkaloids found in the master plant, the first of its kind.

Today, the most active promoter of the healing effects of ayahuasca is a journalist from Britain by the name of Graham Hancock. He talks openly about how consciousness is affected by psychedelics and how human kind has an ancient connection with these healing master plants. He candidly talks about his personal encounters with different types of psychedelic drugs around the world and was featured on TED talk. However, his presentation *The War on Consciousness* was banned for his open discussion about how these plants clearly alter our consciousness in an enlightening way.

Ayahuasca has been used extensively for healing and medicinal purposes for thousands of years. It has been recorded that the Shamans in Peru shared the knowledge of the master plant with the Mestizo holy people to spread the wisdom of care to patients within the Amazon. You will find the Amazonian indigenous communities who have been using ayahuasca for healing and incredible insight mainly in the jungles of Brazil, Ecuador, Colombia and Peru.

During present times, ayahuasca has a more unique use in Brazil as it has been incorporated into the Christian faith. These religious movements of the União do Vegetal and Santo Daime have also found popularity and have spread to establish churches worldwide. They solely use the traditional blend of the master plants and do not combine any admixtures to the brew during their ceremonies.

Quechua is the language spoken in much of the Amazon Basin. It is from two words from this language that the name ayahuasca was created for the vine. "Aya" means *dead* or *soul* and "Huasca" is defined as *rope* or *woody vine*. So the literal translation for ayahuasca is *Vine of Spirits, Vine of the Dead* or *Vine of the Souls.*

Another translation of ayahuasca is the *Rope of the Spirits.* This is due to the link that this vine represents between the spiritual and physical world we live in daily.

The Growing Popularity of Aya

Before the interest in drinking the sacred brew became popular worldwide, you had to venture into the remote areas of South America to participate. Because of the immense desire of Westerners to have this magical experience, there have been countless retreat centers created for this very purpose. The success of the spread of knowledge of ayahuasca has been highly successful and centers are being established all over the globe. The retreats contain the creature comforts and sometimes luxurious settings that were lacking in the traditional ceremonies located in the jungles of the Amazon. However, this opened up the opportunity for many people who did not want to venture into unknown territories alone and created a way for Westerners to receive this medicine in a safe environment.

Because of the spreading knowledge of Ayahuasca, it is being found in places throughout the globe. There has been interest from Westerners who are being initiated in the remote jungles of South America with Shamans to learn the process and have a working relationship with ayahuasca and other teaching plants.

They are following the same initiation process that countless Shamans have learned before them by working with several master plant teachers in addition to ayahuasca to gain knowledge of their healing properties. This has also been a significant measure which has aided the spread of ayahuasca healing throughout the globe as these Western initiates will go on to facilitate ayahuasca ceremonies either back in their home countries or in the retreat centers.

The Amazonian traditions differ so greatly from much of the Western perspective which makes one pay attention to the vastly differing values the Amazonian people believe. Because they are interconnected with the earth and their fellow man, they do not cling onto the finite material items of this world. They have an enlightening perspective on death and also how to live their lives in the most integrated way possible outside of themselves.

When you are partaking in an ayahuasca ceremony, it is important to reflect that this is only one small act that the Amazonian people shamans perform in a grander picture of their lives.

CHAPTER 2

The Science Of Ayahuasca

The Components of Ayahuasca

The ayahuasca vine is comprised of tetrahydroharmine (THH), harmaline and harmine alkaloids. The THH alkaloids are a weak type of serotonin reuptake inhibitor (SRI). THH is responsible for inhibiting the uptake of serotonin in presynaptic neurons and platelets.

The harmaline and harmine alkaloids are the MAOI components which stimulate the central nervous system. The alkaloids also are responsible for ensuring the Dimethyltryptamine, more commonly known by the name of DMT, is not metabolized by the acids in the stomach which aids the substance to be metabolized by the liver instead. When DMT passes the blood-brain barrier, the psychological epiphanies last for several hours and are also the scientific basis for the purging effects you will likely experience.

How Ayahuasca Affects the Brain

The harmaline and harmine alkaloids are quite beneficial for the brain in that they stimulate the release of dopamine which acts as an antidepressant, elevating the individual's mood. It also reduces withdrawal symptoms associated with pain killers and recreational drugs.

They also raise the levels of the brain-derived neurotrophic factor (BDNF) located in the hippocampus section of the brain. The BDNF is responsible for long term memory as well as the development of neurons. There is a famous study that was conducted on the members of the UDV church which concluded that the long term users of ayahuasca had higher than normal levels of brain 5HT transporters. At the time, there was no research related to heightened 5HT levels, they referred to studies that included low levels of the same transporters.

For people who suffer from low 5HT levels, they typically suffer from binge eating, suicidal thoughts, violent behavior and alcoholism. The researchers determined this was from the THH levels that are found in the Aya brew.

The MAOIs are also responsible for curbing cravings and as such as helpful in the matter of addictions that may be experienced by affecting the dopaminergic system.

How the Shamans Work with the Ayahuasca Vine

Madre Ayahuasca is the Mother Spirit of the jungle and governs over all the other spirits of the jungle.

Since the indigenous people of the Amazon work so closely with the sacred plants for a long period of time after their initiation, they are able to recognize the different strains of the ayahuasca vine. They do not follow the Westernized version of taxonomy as they realize this would not be fair to categorize them as such.

This is due to the knowledge they have of the varying strains possessing different healing properties depending on the visions they can induce, the spiritual value of each place, the time they are to be harvested as well as the type of soil in which they are grown. They also identify some of them by the colors of visions that they induce such as yellow, black, white, blue and red.

Others are named by the animals that are likely to be seen such as the monkey, jaguar and boa. Not all the master plants are necessarily visual as they can express themselves through varying senses as we as through extrasensory means. Because the shamans possess such a close connection through the spirits, they can sense all ways in which they communicate.

It may be difficult for some people to believe, but the Amazonian peoples have catalogued approximately 80,000 of the indigenous plants that are found in the jungle. This is a small percentage compared to the estimated one-million more to go. However, they have already categorized this large amount of plants and have an awareness of the healing properties of each, one would have to think about how they were able to acquire such a vast amount of knowledge in a short period of time.

The South American Indian explain that it was Madre Ayahuasca speaking through the vine to guide and educating them on the properties of other master plants that were necessary for healing to occur. With this deep relationship with the vine, trained Shamans would be able to determine the strain of vine from a fair distance and would be able to communicate with the Spirit without ingesting into their system.

Any person with a logical mind would look at the method of trial and error to be quite inefficient when it comes to such a large amount of healing plants.

In traditional cultures, it's often used by shamans or medicine men to open up communication with nature. These spiritual leaders also use it to determine what's causing someone to be sick at the spiritual level.

Shamans use ayahuasca as medicine overall to be able to connect with the energies of nature and to heal psychological wounds. By communicating with the Spirit of the Vine, the Shaman is to gain the knowledge to treat and cure ailments. This also helped them with other community concerns. They also would use the information given by the Spirit of the plant to divine the lover of a person's spouse and who was implementing black magic rituals on members of the community.

Before popularized, the Shaman was the only person to partake during the ceremony to gain guidance as to how to heal people physically and spiritually by being guided by the spirit of the plants. During this time, the members of the community would only drink the concoction once or twice during their lifetimes. This was due to the intense and unpleasant situations that would occur, and they respected the Shaman who had gone through an extensive relationship with the Master Plant to perform the healing work. Now the ceremony has evolved since the explosion of interest in the Vine of the Soul.

To cultivate a relationship with this Master plant, the Shamans would spend an extended duration of time sometimes extending to five years to partake and commune with the Spirit of the Vine as well as other teacher plants to learn of their values and effects. These journeys with these plants were part of the rigorous diet that was to be followed. This aided them to fully be able to use the knowledge that was gained for the betterment of the people, the environment and the community as a whole by being able to ask questions of the Mother Spirit to guide them in their learning.

During this initiation period, the student is creating the plant medicine pharmacy to be able to treat a myriad of illnesses for the members of their community. They spend an ample amount of time with each master plants and trees they are told to work with through Madre Ayahuasca and it an extremely taxing endeavor as it sends the initiate to the very edges or their mental, physical and spiritual capacity. These plants are extremely powerful and the energy that is felt when they are connected fully with them is immense as ayahuasca is not the most potent of all the available master plants. You will have a better insight and appreciation for the Shamans after experiencing ayahuasca's extremely powerful energy for yourself.

They also follow the strict diet which is recommended to participants in the ceremony to gain the full knowledge that Mother Ayahuasca yearns to give. The diet would include no oil, sugar, salt and baked unripened bananas served with white rice. This is in addition to the master plant decoctions. This type of diet is started by the initiate by ingesting cleansing emetics such as *yawarpanga* or sacred tobacco. When they perform these purgatory rites, it is for the same reasoning the shamans will most likely recommend you follow a similar diet before the ceremony. This puts the shaman initiate's body into a state that allows the plant to produce the most benefit.

The Science of Ayahuasca Tea

The creation of the brew takes anywhere from eight hours to a few days depending on the recipe. The basics of the brew preparation include cultivating the *Banisteriopsis caapi* vine, slicing approximately 2 meters of the vine to make one batch of the tea. The branches, leaves and bark are removed and then they are cut into small sections. The pulp is beaten until they are they are fine fibers.

The morning brew is to be made, the leaves of the chacruna are picked and mixed with dried leaves into a large fifty liter boiling pot. They place approximately forty liters of water to cover the master plants and then allow the mixture to slowly boil for about eight hours. They remove the plant matter using a strainer and approximately one liter of the ayahuasca brew remains. One serving of this tea for each participant is approximately two to three ounces.

It takes great care to make this preparation as you can overcook the brew which removes the medicinal properties of the brew. This is a science that the indigenous communities are holding dear. With the tourism business booming, you can find ayahuasca practically anywhere, including roadside stands or markets being sold in simple soda bottles. These road side vendors rope in unsuspecting tourist to buy the supposed brew for nearly $100 which they have no idea who made it, how it was prepared or even if it is authentic.

It is made from a combination of the ayahuasca vine, scientifically known as *Banisteriopsis caapi* and *Psychotria viridis* leaves known by the name of chacruna which translates as *mixture*. There are other medicine plants that certain tribes add to the concoction such as toé or *Brugmansia* and can have differing effects on the participant. There is a specific way the Shamans prepare the brew and the entire process is centered around rituals, singing and creating the space for the Spirit Mother of the Vine and her various other master plant spirits to do her work collectively.

The entheogenic of the brew of ayahuasca is known by different names depending on the area of South America you are partaking. This teacher plant goes by several names including yagé, la purga, la medicina, Aya, caapi, vegetal and daime to name a few.

DMT is the main substance in the chacruna plant which is what is responsible for the psychedelic spiritual encounter with the brewed tea of ayahuasca. DMT is naturally found in animals' brains and in plants naturally. It utilizes serotonin and works with the neural circuits mainly in the frontal cortex, hippocampus and amygdala.

Depending on where the plants are harvested and what time of year, the alkaloid content will differ. Also, the brew itself has a much greater amount of alkaloids than the plants themselves. You will find the average contents of a 200ml cup will be approximately 25 mg DMT, 10 mg THH and 30 mg of harmine/harmaline.

It is believed that the *Psychotria viridis* plant was added to create a higher concentrated emetic to aid in the elimination of parasites in the body. It was found when these two plants were blended that the visionary aspect was impacted greatly than just using the ayahuasca vine on its own.

It is believed that the combination of chacruna was created when the popularity of the healing effects of ayahuasca started to be shared with the world. By all accounts, this is a new development in the ancient history of the indigenous Amazonian peoples as they solely used the ayahuasca vine in their divining rituals for healing.

How Ayahuasca Tea Affects the Brain

When these areas of the brain are affected by the serotonin levels being disrupted in the 5-HT2A receptors, there are huge impacts on the emotional and introspection processing. These are also the same receptors that are activated with other psychedelic drugs such as psilocybin and LSD. Since DMT reacts in your brain much like pharmaceutical SSRIs, the feeling of your mood elevates. The areas of the brain that are affected by DMT are the frontal lobe, pineal gland, hippocampus and amygdala.

The frontal lobe is the part of the brain that is responsible for many different aspects namely consciousness, where the memory banks are stored, the feelings of empathy and communication. The pineal gland is activated while your physical body is left in a vulnerable state which results in an expansion of consciousness and leads to a search deep within ourselves.

The hippocampus is the location where your emotions are stored and is part of the limbic system. It also is where the long-term memory is stored.

The amygdala is also a section of the limbic system that is where one's fears are based along with emotional memory and reactions.

With these areas of the brain being activated, it is obvious why the effects of drinking the brew are based on our past experiences and emotions associated with them.

It has also been discovered that ayahuasca brew significantly reduced the activity in the Default Mode Network (DMN) of the brain. The function of the DMN is how our mind interacts with our surroundings. This can be seen in subjects with traumatic events in their past having a certain reaction to stimuli found in their interpersonal relationships. When events occur that triggers these defaults in the DMN, it acts as a fuel to create cyclical patterns and if left unattended, they can form into mental health disorders.

With ayahuasca showing us the root of the emotions and reactions attached to these traumatic events, it ends up breaking the default within the DMN so that new healthy patterns can be learned. You literally can break the cycle of the hold these traumatic events have held over you.

It also has been proven that the mechanism of ayahuasca promotes mindfulness and detachment from negative thought patterns. This leads partakers to be able to be detached from these previous traumas as well as to be able to approach stressful life scenarios in a healthier way.

When ayahuasca is consumed solely, the visions that occur are shapeless and in black and white. It is through the use of the DMT containing chacruna that the visual display is dramatically heightened.

It is a solidified belief that the natural diet that is followed by the indigenous shamans gives them a heightened sensitivity to DMT. The typical Western diet naturally destroys the DMT molecules naturally present in the brain due to high amounts of monoamine oxidase enzymes being consumed in aged and processed foods.

Because the shamans have acquired this sensitivity to the sole use of ayahuasca, they are able to fine tune their focus on the healing of the ayahuasca vine directly. Westerners are simply not able to receive the same visual benefit from the vine itself, so they combination with chacruna or other admixtures are blended for these individuals to have an experience they can use to heal themselves mentally, physically and spiritually.

The side effects from the DMT that is contained in the ayahuasca vine include increased blood pressure and heart rate, dilated pupils, dizziness and agitation. When you take high amounts of DMT, you will likely experience seizures. The psychological effects include hallucinations and altered perceptions to reality.

The Spiritual Effect of Ayahuasca Tea

The beauty of the Master plant is to bring you in touch with your higher self. It facilitates this connection to bring you the knowledge and insight that is required to gain the guidance to answer the problems that you are facing in your life.

As with everything along spiritual measures, it is not an easy process and you must have the correct intention and respect when taking this avenue to better understanding.

Drinking yagé is not something to do on a whim as it can easily turn your life as you know it upside down. Most people who are not looking for another psychedelic trip to put under their belts has this understanding and goes into the ceremony with respect. As Aya has been referred to as "the most honest mirror" it is hard to take this decision lightly. This is why it is of utmost importance to make sure you are ready to see yourself in that light as it rips your ego apart which makes you feel small in the bigger picture of the Universe yet ultimately connected.

Ayahuasca makes you take a hard look at the beliefs, ideologies, realities and ideas that you use to define yourself and your ego. She shows you who you really are and what that means to you going forward.

Since the spread of the brew, the concoction has been intensified in some cases to bring about profound experiences for Western users. This would explain why certain indigenous communities can take the drink several times a month and not have such an immense reaction to Aya. They are using it is for a different purpose and are using a less potent mixture, if not just pure master plants singularly.

Aside from the medical issues that may be involved, the experience of Ayahuasca is not for every person as it takes you to the extreme boundaries of what you can handle on both sides of the spectrum. For the casual user who is researching for their first retreat may shy away from their decision at this point. This is for the best as the vine needs to be respected for the medicine that it is used for and is not a cure-all for anything physical, mental or spiritual that you are going through. Even though you may have a profound indescribable experience, you still need to put the effort into making sure the communion with Mother Aya is not in vain.

When you feel like you have lost the connection with the world around you, Shamanism may be the answer you start to delve into. When we think of healing Shamans, they are connected with their inner and outer worlds with a deep understanding of the energies of both worlds.

Using plants to heal and teach is a way of life for people of the Amazon rainforest. The plants themselves can become your travel companions as you journey towards a more complete version of yourself. As we walk this path, the teacher plants heal and guide much like a best friend and they like to remind you that all life is sacred and holy.

The plants are able to heal because they are the direct source of powerful energy from Mother Earth. You are able to embody their immense power when the playground of your physical and subtle body energy is clear.

The voice of the Spirit is of feminine nature which is why she is referred to as the Mother Spirit. She speaks through the master plant to direct you on the areas that need attention in your life to facilitate you achieving your goals.

If you are feeling you are being drawn to have your own lesson from Mother Aya, then you likely will find She will find you. She will plant a seed of awareness in your consciousness, and your path will automatically lead you to where you are to experience Her.

How Admixtures Affect the Tea

In some indigenous communities, they have admixtures which combine other stimulants into the mix. This is not always a good combination for first time users of the brew. This is due to participants not having a tolerance compared to the indigenous peoples who partake regularly and these admixtures differentiate in intensity depending on the time of year they are harvested which affects the amounts of alkaloids contained within.

Beware that many times there are other admixtures to the brew that you may not even be aware have been blended with the tea. Be sure to inquire about the exact ingredients at the ceremony that you are attending so that you are completely aware of what you are putting into your body. The ceremony may take a much different turn with these admixtures involved. If your facilitator is honest and forthcoming with this information, then there should be nothing to worry about as they are the experts and you need to trust them.

There are several common admixtures that are used in ayahuasca brews. These are in addition to any other purging plants that are given by certain Shamans to clear the body of blockages. Remember to inquire further with your Shaman about the uses, benefits and side effects so you are aware of what may be experienced during and after the ceremony. Here is a brief overview.

- Remo Caspi bark (*Aspidosperma excelsum*) removes dark and dense energies in the subtle body energy. Medicinal use is mainly for malaria. However other uses are for cancer, diabetes, inflammation, high blood pressure, hepatitis, digestive disorders and fevers.
- Tamamuri (*Brosimum acutifolium*) is a protector and wards off the energies that are removed from the participants. Medicinal uses are blood purifier, inflammation, anti-parasitic, fungal infections, cancer, arthritis, syphilis and antibacterial.
- Chullachaki Caspi bark (*Byrsonima christianeae*) is a purgatory plant that also aids in transcending ailments of the physical body.
- Capirona bark (*Calycophyllum spruceanum*) gives protections and cleaning. Medicinal uses include treatment for eye infections, fungal infections on the skin and is an anti-diabetic.
- Huacapurana (*Campsiandra angustifolia*) provide grounding during the ceremony. Medicinal uses include malaria, fever, diarrhea, arthritis and Lyme's disease.
- Wyra Caspi bark (*Cedrelinga caeniformis*) brings tranquility and calms the mind. Also to relieve the body of intestinal and gastric ailments by the act of purging.

- Lupuna Blanca bark (*Ceiba pentandra*) gives protection. Medicinal uses include Type II diabetes, headaches and diuretic.
- Ayahuma bark (*Couroupita guianensis*) gives protection and heals the soul that was lost from spiritual trauma or fright. Medicinal uses include malaria, stomach ache, inflammation, pain, tumors and hypertension.
- Shiwawaku bark (*Dipteryx odorata)* gives protection. Medicinal uses are anti-parasitic and diarrhea.
- Camu camu Gigante (*Myrciaria dubia)* keeps demonic spirits and dark energies at bay. Medicinally treats cardiovascular ailments, some cancers, diabetes and arthritis.
- Uchu sanango (*Tabernaemontana sanaango*) gives strength, power and protection. Medicinally it is used for opiate addictions and pain management. The main alkaloid in this plant is iboga which is a psychoactive compound which naturally occurs. It also gives the same side effects of spiritual exploration and psychological introspection as ayahuasca.
- Punga Amarilla bark gives protection by removing negative energies in the subtle body energy.

Warnings about Admixtures

Beware of the admixture of 5-MeO-DMT also known by the name of *anadenanthera pilgrim*, *yopo* or *cohaba*. This substance is most known to cause serotonin syndrome and interact negatively with harmaline and harmine which are found in the ayahuasca vine. The side effects closely mimic those found in the ayahuasca vine. Shamans use yopo to enhance the effects of the ayahuasca tea. When mixed incorrectly, added adverse side effects are long term kidney damage, seizures, elevated blood pressure, heart rate and temperature and, in extreme cases, death.

The admixture related to 5-MeO-DMT is *virola theiodora* also known as red virola which also contains DMT. This is used by the South American Shamans as a snort and also, scarily, as arrow poison. The side effects are hallucinations, lucid dreams, dream states, headache and dizziness.

Toé (*Brugmansia)* is a hallucinogenic which heightens the visionary encounter through the alkaloids of atropine and scopolamine. A very small amount of this admixture is all that is required as it is extremely potent and have a more vivid encounter with Mother Ayahuasca. On the other hand, it is potentially dangerous if mixed incorrectly. Overdose side effects of toé include convulsions, temporary loss of sight, dehydration, poisoning, seizures, dilated pupils, hyperventilation, amnesia, delirium, life-like hallucinations, unconsciousness and even death in extreme cases.

Finally, use extreme caution with the admixture of *bufo alvarius* which comes from the Colorado River and Sonora Desert toad. This is the toxic venom that is secreted from their skin and has started to be infused into ayahuasca tea. Overdose side effects of this admixture are permanent paralysis, seizures and death.

The Male Counterpart

San Pedro (*Echinopsis pachanoi)* is also known by the name of Wachuma and is a cactus master plant.

It is the masculine counterpart to ayahuasca and as such is the opposite. However, there are many similarities that bind these two master plants in a special way where they work together beautifully.

San Pedro is said to give you the strength and courage to carry out what you have learned through Mother Ayahuasca. It also is able to give you a consciousness expansion along with prophecies.

The ceremonies are usually held during the day whereas the ceremonies for ayahuasca are held generally at night time. There are no intense visions or the purge effect with this cactus. There is an immense opening of the heart chakra that occurs after drinking the slimy concoction which allows for you to heal your past wounds in a positive way.

It even goes as deep to heal the very diseases and psychological injuries in your DNA.

The effects last for at least fourteen hours and usually you can still feel the medicine in your system through the next morning. The ceremonies are more upbeat with many drums and songs because this master plant has a more outward expression.

Mescaline is the main alkaloid in this cactus and can be used to treat depression and alcoholism. The side effects which can be less intense than ayahuasca are colorful visual effects, the loss of the concept of time as well as altered perceptions and thinking process.

Like ayahuasca, Wachuma will bring imprinted beliefs and past traumas to the surface to have you face them in a heartfelt way. It also has the effect of ego death where you feel the interconnectedness with the Universe.

If you would like to experience the whole spectrum of these complementary master plants, it will not be a difficult task to be able to find a shaman that specializes in ceremonies for both of these teachers. Many times San Pedro ceremonies are offered with the same Shamans who conduct the ayahuasca ceremonies, especially at retreat centers.

CHAPTER 3

Ayahuasca Ceremonies

Shaman or a Charlton?

The Shamans are called by different names depending on the region they were born. For example, the Amazonian Shamans are known by the name of Shipibo *ayahuasqueros* or *Onanya*s whereas the Shamans from the Andean Mountains are referred to as a *Q'ero Paqos*. Most indigenous communities do not even call them Shamans as they are the local doctors who protect and heal and are known commonly as *medicos*.

When choosing your Shaman, have a conversation with them first and shy away from anyone who has a website or directly comes to you to offer you the drink. True Shamans of ayahuasca are quiet spoken and humble. You may not even realize that they are Shamans in the first place as they are not in the limelight. You will find that true Shamans are well adapted members of their society. They have a stable life and usually have a family. When they are mysterious and solitary, this is a sign that they probably do not have the right intentions.

Through the years of rigorous training, they have dealt with their own demons within by going to Hell and back. By taking you into their sacred space of the ceremony, they are agreeing to make sure that if you are found in the same difficult position that they will come to the same space energetically to bring you out.

Without saying, the Shamans should gain the same respect as you give to the Master plant herself.

When a healer starts on their path working with Madre Aya and being initiated as a student of shamanism, they are given a tool of magical darts known as *tsentsak*. They receive these during their initiation into this path and have to choose the light or dark path of which to use them. These darts are just like they sound. They penetrate into the subtle energy body and can cause blockages to create illness, spiritual obstacles or even death. When the initiated Shaman to be receives the tsentsak, they are challenged with mastering their desires to use these for a higher purpose and thus gains the knowledge in how to heal others.

Considering all people have choices, this does not exclude the holy Shamans as they have to continuously chose to use their divining powers for the better good of nature and the community. They can always go to the "dark side" by becoming witch doctors and casting spells and curses as well. You must be diligent and follow your intuition when it comes to choosing the person you are going to need to fully trust during the ceremony.

There are people outside of the indigenous communities as well as within who are taking the opportunity to take advantage sexually and ethically of unsuspecting people. This is especially true in places where travelers and backpackers frequent looking to experience the awakening. In these cases, the traditional rituals are not precise as to what the original experiences were in the secluded jungles of the Amazon and more often than not, they are separated entirely from the practices that were performed for thousands of years.

Keep an eye out for so called healers who obviously have psychological issues or addictions themselves including alcoholism. This also includes pride and boasting about their powers. They may even be criminals who have no knowledge in the ways of shamanism and will cause you ill harm physically to get what they desire. These so called shamans may give you what seems like ayahuasca tea, but it will have little if no effect on you. On the other hand, it can put into a state that makes you unaware of your surroundings which would make you vulnerable.

Because of this, you must research to make sure you are being supervised by a properly trained Shaman who has gone through the rigorous training to deserve the title. You want to ensure that you have a knowledgeable and trustworthy person who will be able to guide you properly through the dark areas that Ayahuasca can take you as well as explain the other beautiful experiences that you participate in so that you can take the information that Mother Ayahuasca gives you to make the most of the experience.

There are not as many highly trained Shamans as you may think because roughly twenty percent of the initiates reach the final stage of their journey. This shows that there are many people out there who have gone through the path of learning about these master plants. However, there are going to be more who have just gained some information but not all and this is quite dangerous when it comes to working with someone on the energetic and spiritual scale that ayahuasca provides. So of course they will be knowledgeable on some degree, but just like you reading about the knowledge in this book, this in no way makes you a Shaman.

Many people may end up assuming that these Shamans are fully enlightened. Some may be by the Western definition. However, the viewpoint and belief system of the Amazonian healers differs much from Western thought as they are more connected to nature than we ever could be with the modernization and technology of the Western world. This is how they have learned to live in the versatile environment of the Amazon and have passed these ideals down through the generations to be able to survive through dangerous scenarios such as monsoon like rains, dark magic from sorcerers, evil entities, poisonous plants and creatures, and diseases.

The Shamans you want to work with will have had a relationship with Aya for at least 10 years. This way you can be assured they have seen all types of situations and have a firm understanding of ayahuasca under their belts. For a better sense of trust of the Shaman's knowledge, inquire about their lineage and who was their teacher. When they speak of these people, it should be in a humble and honor driven manner without boastfulness.

The true Shamans are the beings that can transcend the urge to harm others while they are in this incapacitating state after partaking in ayahuasca tea. Because they have taken the rigorous training to heal through Mother Ayahuasca, they have developed an immense dedication to not use their channeling powers for evil. If they are not capable of doing this, they simply are a sorcerer or witch doctor who has no discipline or self-control. This is a harder task than you would think because surprisingly the darker path of harming people is much easier than taking the path of healing.

If you are dealing with a dark healer, they can manipulate you in ways you would not realize and cause physical and psychological harm. Just the opposite of a true healing Shaman, they can create illnesses within your body and mind as well as have you possessed by demons and evil spirits. When a doctor takes this path, it is mainly due to the lack of experience with Spirit and them not possessing the will power which is necessary for the line of work they are performing. This is the very reason you must be diligent in vetting the Shaman you will be working with and trusting on every level of your being.

When a Shaman has the true path of healing others and the environment around them, they possess a high level of desire to use their powers for the highest level of betterment. When they continue on this path, they are granted more gifts through the Master plant spirits and expand on their channeled healing gifts.

There are thousands of Master Plants that are used as a medicine to treat past emotional and traumatic instances, psycho-spiritual ailments as well as energetic imbalances. The understanding of the Amazon Shaman traditions is that the Spirit of the Ayahuasca vine is the mother of all the Master plants and controls the other master plants beneath her. She shares with the Shaman the powerful healing knowledge these specific plants have. The Shaman then acts as a channel to work the will of the Master plants by healing their patients.

Because the Amazonian life is so interconnected with nature and the spirits found within, Shamans have a keen eye for imbalances around them. They instinctively know the difference between light and dense energies and who are malevolent and benevolent spirits. They use this awareness to call upon different master plants that are needed for the type of ceremony that is to be performed.

If you have found a Shaman to work with, take the time to sit with them as much as you can before making the decision to trust him completely. Use your intuition and question them with any inquiries. They should be forthcoming with answers for all your questions and not deflect to divert your attention from your original line of questioning. The true Shamans are transparent, protective and want to have an open environment in which everyone feels comfortable in the space.

How Much Does a Ceremony Cost

There is a varying range of costs that are associated with going to a ceremony with an individual Shaman who is working on their own versus going to an all-inclusive retreat center as you can expect. If you are able to find an indigenous Shaman within their own communities, the costs are going to range from $35 to $60 for each ceremony you attend. The costs to be able to stay for up to a week will run you approximately $400 and usually a meal a day is included in this price. You will also get to have the true experience of the Amazon while you are in the small indigenous communities.

When you go through a retreat center which is much more involved with preparation and integration sessions range from $800 to $2000 for a week long stay. This includes your food, having facilitators available for any questions that arise as well as spa services such as saunas, swimming pools and massages. They also usually have extensive security for their center so you feel safer.

The Breakdown of the Ceremony

Even with the ever growing popularity of the Aya brew ceremonies, it has been found that the ritual itself is a fairly new development in the history of the South American Indian Shaman medicine work. However, they have been using the Mother Vine to assist in giving direction for healings as well as medicine itself.

The main place where the indigenous tribes who perform the ceremonies are found in the Amazon Basin in the northwest section. Specifically, where Brazil, Ecuador, Peru and Columbia join together. There are also groups of Mestizo communities that have a strong hold in Pucallpa and Iquitos in Peru. However, you can find the ceremony throughout the world held underground as DMT is a Schedule I controlled substance which makes it illegal to possess outside of a religious context.

There are three types of ceremonies that you will come in contact with: the traditional shaman ceremony, the therapeutic ceremony or religious ceremony.

All the ceremonies will include the facilitator or Shaman guiding you through the entire process before, during and after. It usually is conducted during the night as there are less distractions from daily life during this time. However, there are instances where the ceremony is conducted during the daytime. Getting yourself in touch with the understanding and master intelligence which is within every human being. You very well will get in touch with the creator of all that you know and is going to be a journey to places you cannot imagine or conceive.

There are several people who are officially able to conduct the ceremonies. They can be a padrinho, therapist, healer or a Mestre if going to the ayahuasca churches.

Ayahuasca sessions are usually done in a group setting ranging from five to twenty-five people; occasionally, there may be as many as one hundred participants in a session—or even more.

The Shaman is also present to maintain order and peace in the space. He is in charge of all the people to ensure that negative energies are dissipated through the assistance of the called upon spirits and to heighten the energy of the space when required through the *icaros*. To ensure the participants are present, cell phones and other electronics are not allowed in this sacred space as they would be distracting to yourself and other participants.

The deaths that have been reported for users of Aya are directly related to them not following instructions of the Shaman. This includes continuing to imbibe in drugs, alcohol and nicotine before the ceremony as well as undiagnosed physical conditions. You will find many retreat centers will require you to have a recent full health screen to ensure your safety during the ceremonies.

The shaman or a designated facilitator will ritually prepare the ayahuasca tea the day of the ceremony. There are retreat centers that have other people make the medicine and then have it transported to the site as well. It depends on the team of experts they have on hand at the center.

Traditional Shaman Ceremony

The Shaman, neo-shaman or Vegetalistas are the names of the people who run these traditional ceremonies. They are the most important integral part of the ceremony as they are in control of creating a safe space for the Ayahuasca Spirit and other master plant spirits to work as well as healing you on an emotional and psychological level. Utmost trust needs to be processed for the Shaman as you may find yourself in some extremely disturbing or enlightening experiences that you will need a guiding hand.

Sometimes you are asked to bathe in natural areas or with certain plants before the ceremony to ensure you are properly cleansed before starting. If you take a trip to the Amazon, you will most certainly be outdoors under an open sided building with only a roof known as a *maloka* so that you can easily commune with nature.

There are other shamans who believe in performing the purging and cleansing of the body before the ceremony begins by using sacred tobacco leaves called *mapacho* to induce the purging effect. When you arrive at the ceremony, you are able to focus more on the journey rather than suffering through the purge the entire time. This act of purging beforehand minimizes the amount of purging that occurs with the ayahuasca tea.

It is absolutely recommended to get yourself in a clear state of mind before starting the ceremony. You are encouraged to focus on your breathing or perform meditation to center and prepare your mind. These ceremonies are focused on spiritual encounters and healing oriented, and helps to be in a good space in your heart and mind before entering.

When the ceremony begins, there may be a time for all the participants to share their intention. The Shaman will then bless the tea before serving individually to everyone at the ceremony. He invokes protection against negative energies and inputs a conduit for the spirits to use the tea for their healing energies by blowing the sacred mapacho tobacco smoke into the tea. He will also use Agua Florida or Palo Santo incense to consecrate the mixture. They will then call for all the participants to form a line to commence the dispensing of the brew.

From all accounts, the brew has a very bitter and earthy taste and is not something that will be enjoyed if sipped. It is best to quickly swallow the mixture and be sure to keep yourself from vomiting for a minimum of 15 minutes so that the concoction can properly integrate into your system.

You will find if you are going to drink more than once that the first dose will be smaller to get your body accustomed to the medicine as well as to establish a relationship with the vine. This is also to make sure that your journey is not thrown into a high sensory mode which makes it difficult to deal with certain situations during your first session. It is best to take these things slow as they will take time to digest.

After all the participants drank, the Shaman will partake and make the space dark by blowing out any candles that are being used. You are free to roam about if needed, but you will be urged to lay down quietly on a mat that is provided for you so that you can sink into this silent space. Usually there are other items to make you comfortable during the ceremony to include towels and pillows. You may also be given plant infused water to keep your hydration levels high.

The stage where you start to feel the effects of the brew is known as *mareacion* and takes you into the fourth dimension which has you in contact with the differing plant spirits. Sometimes the Shaman will bring in as many as forty teaching plant spirits to aid in the healing during the session. These plant spirits work through the Shaman to ensure the space is cleaned of negative energies as well as protected.

Their presence is paramount to the ceremony as the spirit plants work with Madre Ayahuasca who in turn works through the Shaman to facilitate the space for the causes of disease, trauma and imbalances to emerge energetically.

When approximately half an hour passes, the effects of the Ayahuasca will start to be apparent and the Shaman will start to sing the icanos to bring your consciousness into a space to enhance the visions that Mother Ayahuasca is going to give you.

These chants and songs are specific to different master plants as they are being called to enter the sacred space of the ceremony to aid in the enhancement of the visions and connection you will receive. There is also an icano for Mother Ayahuasca who is brought in to be the master of all the other plant spirits during the ceremony. There may just be the chants that the shaman sings or the facilitators may incorporate drums, mouth harp or maracas into the space.

By the time the music starts, you should start to feel the medicine starting to crawl through your body much like a snake. It will make you feel a tug of war between cold chills and fever and you may start to feel the purge of the negativity begin to rise.

For the purpose of purging, there are usually small pots left by your space and tissue for using the restroom or wiping your mouth. It is not a pretty situation, but the release is well worth it after it is complete as your mind will become more clear and calm. Mother Ayahuasca will be able to do her best.

In the meantime, you start to drift into a state which is very dream like yet based in reality. It may seem like a life end review with how many thoughts and images that come into your mind. Some people even lay down and experience a state between waking and sleeping that is very vivid and surreal.

Once the medicine starts to do Her work, you will start to lose the sense of time and your body my morph into various animals or you may see them around other participants. Remember to keep in mind to not be afraid and to continue to stay open no matter how unbelievable what you are witnessing.

The common way that Spirit comes through to you is as an anaconda. You may feel as if you are being strangled at first as She is integrating into your body. You can start communicating fully with her at that time. Once she is fully blended inside of you, this is the moment that you let go of everything that frightens you about the situation as then you will have the most enlightening experience.

At certain times during the ceremony, the Shaman may blow tobacco smoke or Palo Santo incense to alter the sacred space to push the partakers in different directions during the journey. This method is known by the name of *soplar* and may achieved while he is sitting at his place or by coming by to do this individually for each participant. You may have a facilitator or the Shaman themselves come to you to quietly interact during the ceremony. There are also instances that certain shamans will come to you individually to aid in the master plant work personally. The Shamans remove the dense energies from the participant by performing *chupar* by sucking the energy out of the participant in addition to the method of *soplar*.

Over the course of approximately 4 to 6 hours, you will be drifting in and out of this dreamlike state whether you are sitting up and aware or laying down seemingly asleep. However, your consciousness is quite awake and taking all the information like a sponge. The medicine helps you to see yourself and the things that you have done in an objective light. This is the way to fully release the bonds these memories have on you and to go forward with this information acting in a more beneficial way for all involved.

Even though all ceremonies differ depending on your location and beliefs of that Shaman facilitating, they typically last anywhere from 2 to 4 days. The ceremonies themselves are anywhere from three to 7 hours long.

The Shaman may start dancing while singing the icaros as everyone sits in a circle around a fire. The fire is a cleansing aspect as well as a way for the Shaman to observe each participate during the ceremony to determine if he needs to change the mood with a different icaros, sacred incense or if an individual needs specific care.

There are different requirements during the ceremony depending on the Shaman. They may welcome you to sing along with him or expect you to stay in a quiet space to fully take in the experience. These are ground rules which will be understood before the ceremony begins. If not, be sure to ask what the protocol is for your specific ritual.

While the Shaman is singing, he is conversing with the spirits of the Master Plants to guide and heal the participants on a deep level. He is working with the whole team of master plant spirits as they are all needed in conjunction with the Spirit of Aya to carry out the highest intention for all those involved in the ceremony. When you have a thoroughly trained Shaman, they are able to carry out all of these tasks simultaneously while keeping an eye on each individual's energy.

If the Shaman notices that you need personal attention but is not able to stop the multiple tasks he is performing, he will have his organizers come to help.

The ceremonies take place at night because most of the jungle spirits are sleeping and you will be able to communicate with the Spirit of the Vine more clearly.
After the ceremony, the Shaman will likely perform a ritual to clean each individual who participated. This is to rid them of any residual negative energy that may be present in the subtle energy body. These energies are attracted to them because of the state of vulnerability they were in.
It is most common to wear white during the ceremony.

Therapeutic Ceremony

These ceremonies are a bridge between the traditional ceremonies and Western psychotherapy. These sessions are based more on personal growth process and use ayahuasca as a therapeutic tool. There may be possibilities of one on one work during these sessions and can last for upwards to a month's time to be able to address the entire scope of healing. Each ceremony would have a period that would involve preparation for the drinking of ayahuasca as well as a phase of integration.
The fashion these ceremonies vary greatly and depend upon who is facilitating the ceremonies. They are more modern in the sense that they do not just chant songs. They like to blend silence, live and digital music into the sessions.
With the therapeutic approach, they are looking at a more Western style of healing which includes massages and sauna sessions. You will also likely bathe with plants and flowers.
If you are specifically going for medical treatment through ayahuasca, you will likely be given many types of master plants to work with over the duration of time you will be there to fully give you the chance to heal inside and out.
If you are looking for a more integrated approach to self-healing in a therapeutic setting, this is the way to go. It is more hands on and intensive overall as there are many opportunities to work through your issues on multiple platforms compared to a traditional Shamanic ceremony which may or may not have group integration periods.

A therapeutic ceremony is also recommended for those who are seeking to rid themselves of destructive behavioral issues as well as release themselves from traumatic events.

Religious Ceremonies

Religious Ceremonies are centered around the União do Vegetal and Santo Daime churches. They focus on drinking ayahuasca multiple times a month and have the Christian/Catholic aspect blended into the experience. There are also instances where there are healing sessions as well. The ceremonies are very structured and ritualized and have a focus point of unity with the works in the community. As expected, they sing hymns during the ceremonies interspersed with durations of time that you can reflect in silence.

There may be instances in which the members are able to have open questions to the Mestres about their religious and philosophical issues. Other forms of ceremonies include simple dances in which the participants participate. There usually is not an integration session included in the ceremony. Because these churches are found in small communities, especially in Brazil, the members all keep in contact with each other. This creates a buddy system of checking up on the spiritual progress of each other.

Tips to Assist During the Ceremony

While going on the journey using the brew as a facilitator, you are able to answer the greatest questions that all human beings ask: What is my purpose? Who is God and is there one? Why are here living this experience on earth? Why am I going through this situation? How can I live my life better?

We usually only gain understanding of these concepts during near-death experiences or near the brink of death. We gain all the knowledge that was contained within ourselves all along. And with the aid of ayahuasca, you can start remembering this knowledge and be able to apply it in your life when it is most useful.

The overall experience that you encounter will directly be related to the amount of work you put in ahead of time.

Because of the spiritual nature of this Master plant, it should be respected as Mother Nature herself because this is what the Shamans thoroughly believe. You must seek supervision as you are put into a state of immobility in most instances and may go through disturbing experiences such as your own ego death which may end badly without the correct guidance. There are also instances where fainting has occurred, so it best to be sitting or lying down during the experience.

Some people who are interested in drinking the brew for the first time seem to be drawn to the psychedelic experiences they will obtain from the DMT found within the vine. However, this is the wrong approach. Madre Ayahuasca needs to be addressed with utmost respect and reverence as the Shamans practice in their daily lives. The Spirit of the vine is an excellent teacher and is willing to guide the individual who has an open mind who surrenders to Her.

The ceremony should not be taken lightly and you should always possess the highest respect for the Master plant and the Shaman facilitators. The amount of energy that you personally put into the ceremony beforehand will also determine the outcome during and after the ceremony. It cannot be stressed enough that a positive, forgiving and understanding mindset is the best during your journey with ayahuasca.

Sometimes there are other master plants or *mapacho*, sacred tobacco, that is smoked by the participants. Make sure you have a clear understanding how your specific ceremony is going to be held and what to expect ahead of time so you can ask questions if you have any.

Make sure that you know the entire schedule for rest days or if you are needing to leave the space immediately. Sometimes the facilitators and Shaman is available afterwards for the integration session to be able to talk about your experiences and to get an insight into the visions you were not able to decipher on your own. Some participants believe they should keep these encounters between them and the Shaman as it is their sacred knowledge and only for them. Other retreat centers believe in sharing the integration session with the entire group to help each other understand their own personal experiences.

During the tough and dark times of the ceremony, bring yourself back to your center by focusing on your breathing and take conscious, deep breaths to bring you back to your purpose of bringing you here. Your intention must be strong and heartfelt as this will be your ultimate guide to getting through these tougher times of the ceremony.

The purging which will occur is not like any other time you have been ill. Because it is an intense spiritual cleaning, the experience will be likewise. If you find the thought of purging in front of others and sharing the vulnerability of the situation, then it you may want to rethink about taking the medicine because in all honesty, there are more intense sections of the ceremony that you will likely experience. Once you have surrendered to this simple fact, you are able to see the bigger picture as to why you are here.

If you are finding the visions to be too intense, the trick is to open your eyes and scan around you. This will not take the visions completely away, but rather make them slightly less intense. Remember these are your personal lessons and it is important to not shy away from the mirror that is being placed before you. It will give you the insight as to why you decided to come in the first place.

When you are transported to visualizing other dimensions, you need to certainly let go of expectations. There are no rules or time in these places and anything can happen.

If you are given the opportunity to drink a second helping of the brew, make sure that you are still in the proper mindset to be on the journey. Every body soaks up the medicine differently and it may take a while for you to feel the effects. You may be setting yourself up for a double dose to come on rather quickly once taking the second drink. However, if you are already in the vision state of the ceremony, it will continue to elevate the deepening of the experience.

Do not get frustrated if you do not have certain effects come to you during your experience, especially if this is your first time with Aya. Know that the Master plant is much more intelligent and realizes what she is doing. This is why you need to trust her and not have any expectations of your personal experience going into the ceremony.

No matter how much research or preparation you think you have achieved, you will be unprepared for the event. But by keeping your focus on your intention of what led you to Ayahuasca - or what she led you to - will get you the knowledge and insight required to realize those intentions.

When the visions become less intense, the effects of the brew are starting to wear off.

There is no way to prepare for the darker aspects of ayahuasca such as when painful and traumatic events in your subconscious emerge other than to simply let go. Your ego will start to react in its instinctual anxiety and fear, but know that this is a temporary feeling and situation. It is not a permanent state of being and will pass.

When you receive your portion of the brew, you may start to doubt such a small amount of liquid could produce such profound results. You may also start to doubt the process after drinking the liquid as it can be quite foul. Put these things out of our mind and focus on the bigger picture of the gift you are about to be given. Once the process is started, there is no other choice other than to see it through to the end.

It is also wise to speak to Mother Ayahuasca as you are receiving the brew. Asking for guidance, repeating your intention to her and asking for her protection and grace. This will show your respect and humility towards her as well as showing your openness to what she is about to show you. Trust in your Shaman and yourself at this point as well. Know in your heart that you are determined to face yourself to be able to understand the best way to go forward physically, mentally and spiritually. Then continue to focus and breath as you feel the medicine flowing through your body, scanning for any blockages and places that need the most attention. This is a rite of passage that you owe to yourself and the people you surround yourself with in your daily life.

You may also feel like you have flu like symptoms or even food poisoning as well as finding it difficult to move or walk about. This is nothing to be worried about as it will soon pass. Just find a comfortable position to sit or lay until the feeling passes. Remember to go with the flow as you are located in this sacred, healing space which is safe and protected.

The process uncovers the ultimate knowledge that you already possess that you have gained throughout your lifetime, but you have forgotten. It removes what makes you ill physically and mentally through the purge and enlightens you with what you must connect with to be healthy. It lightens the baggage you carry around with you, conscious and unconscious. It brings understanding of the suffering of the Universe yet rises you to the utmost joy. If you come in with an open and surrendering heart, you will walk away with a profound encounter.

It helps you to understand the darkness as well as the light. You must put your faith in whatever you hold dear while you walk through the darkness and know that this is where the true wisdom of yourself lies. Once the thoughts and feelings that you have been hiding from emerge, you can confront them knowing that you will never need to ever think of these things ever again. You have learned your lesson and can go forward without the weight on your shoulders and with gratitude in your heart. You mind will be amazingly clear with your purpose and path you need to follow in this life.

The music is an integral aspect of spiritual ceremonies. Incorporating songs into spiritual journeys has been occurring for thousands of years because there is actually a purpose behind them. Even science has proven this with studies showing through brain scans that certain areas of the brain are activated depending on the wanted outcome. So welcome the music as it can be a welcome distraction and focus point when you are going through the rougher patches of your journey.

Many of the deaths and negative outcomes that have been reported are due to lack of supervision, not following the diet recommendations, known & unknown physical conditions and not reporting prescription drugs you have been taking. It is imperative that you must be honest with the Shaman conducting the ceremony about these things as he will know if it is appropriate for you to participate or may alter the ceremony to suit your personal needs.

What Experiences to Expect

There are many facets and phases to the experience of ayahuasca and should not be thought of in a linear fashion. Try to see the whole experience as a mini lifetime.

You are going to experience feelings of euphoria as well as sadness. You will also have moments of epiphanies and also disappointment. These are all things that people encounter at one point of their lives. If the experience is too much for you to handle, get the help of the facilitators to help guide you through. After all, they are there to help you to attain the most you can from the session.

A common occurrence while going through the experience is to have long forgotten memories brought back to the surface. This is initiated by Mother Ayahuasca to help us to see the things that we have done in an objective light. What you experience after drinking the tea is extremely personal.

Within about a half hour after consuming ayahuasca tea, people experience something that they describe as hallucinations. People who have used it do not feel like it's the same as a trip they might get with LSD, however, and they describe it as more emotional and spiritual, as opposed to being recreational.

Because the literal translation of Ayahuasca is the vine of death, many times it may feel as if you are on the brink of death or even experience your own ego death. It is much like the Hindu God Shiva who is the destroyer of illusion. It brings you in front of a mirror of anything you have ever thought, said or done. However, this does rely on your intention and the openness that you approach this sacred plant.

It will be a more powerful experience the more you are willing to let go of control and allow the spirit of the plant to take you on a journey. There will be things that will be quite unpleasant as we as a whole are not as pure as we were when we were children. We have made mistakes. We have hurt people. Everything must come to the surface and be faced head on for us to properly let go and rise spiritually as we let go of our own egos.

Even with this said, even with people who have experienced the hard truth about themselves, they feel a sense of relief and calm after the event. You can experience periods of confusion and placement in this world afterwards as your ego is shattered but this is something that some people seek. Awakening and Enlightenment.

The process is difficult to attain true enlightenment, but it is well worth the journey. Once you realize the truth of the illusion, you will have no fear to hold you back. You will make major life changing decisions, but they will not be as grueling as they had been before. You will have a purpose and understanding of your place in this world.

There is a myriad of symptoms that can occur but know that each person's journey is different. You may see vivid and unimaginable alternate dimensions, animals and plant life that seem surreal or family members dead and alive. There have even been accounts of individuals conversing with Mother Ayahuasca herself, obtaining the guidance that they needed to jump over the hurdles in their lives.

Many times, the visions and communication with Spirit cannot be described as you are connecting with the infinite which cannot be fully explained by the compartmental brains we possess. There have also been cases of metaphysical powers such as precognition or telepathy to occur in partakers of the ayahuasca brew.

The information that you receive from you higher power is going to be the catalyst to the greatest changes in your life and is usually not what we expect going in. The best approach is to have no expectations to the outcome and be open to where the journey takes you. You may not like what you see and hear as this is the ultimate true mirror of who you are inside. It taps into your consciousness on the deepest levels and puts you in touch with memories or aspects of yourself that you have forgotten or chose to ignore. When given this clarity, it is up to the individual of how they will use it to change their life for the greater good.

If you happen to partake in Aya more than once, it will more than likely be a different experience. Think of each journey as taking a layer of an onion off piece by piece because no one could go straight to the center and be able to comprehend. There are also multiple layers to the lessons that Madre Ayahuasca has to share with you which all need to be reflected upon before moving even deeper.

The ceremony is intense and has commonly been referred to as a decade worth of therapy during one journey with Her. There is much to learn about ourselves and the world as a whole through the supreme knowledge of Aya. Because of the deep processing that is necessary after drinking, it is extremely important to give yourself the time after the properly dissect and apply the knowledge given to you before considering doing the ceremony again.

The medicine does continue to work after the hallucinogenic effects wear off, and some argue that it never ends. It truly is a life changing experience for many who have chosen the journey.

The mental and emotional aspects will be addressed by bringing unconscious or repressed memories back into the forefront so that they can be seen with a different set of eyes with an objective perspective. This is the ideal time to notice the recurring patterns in our life that have been holding you back from being fulfilled.

You will likely experience the oneness with everything and everyone around you during the ceremony which may bleed into your daily life afterwards. You will be able to have an objective perception of the illusions this world is full of and have a greater understanding of the reasoning behind all that is. The world will not be a boring place but take on an idea of a playground which you can take part in.

You may feel as if you are having a bout of schizophrenia as your mind may not be able to process everything that you are sensing throughout your body as your mind tries to grasp the infinite wisdom you are being gifted. The world as you know it will be an illusion along with your ego and then it will start to build itself back together in a proper way.

This is not a simple process and must be approached in a deep and meaningful way. Before the ceremony, humbly connect with Mother Ayahuasca, creating your intention for the ceremony if you have not already. Talk with the vine and let her know what you are seeking and show your respect for the opportunity to experience this healing event. Prepare your mind to be in a vulnerable state and welcome this feeling.

Any trepidation to the idea will mean you will need to put more energy into the process while will impede the flow. Without the correct mindset, you may not be able to handle the truth of yourself reflecting back at you. Again, leave all expectations at the door. If you had done extensive research and read about other people's experiences ahead of time, leave those behind as well. You will experience what is personal to you. You may have some overlap in what other partaker's have experienced, but it is personalized to you solely.

It is important to know why you are coming to the ceremony will likely be addressed. Any unhealed wounds and traumas will come up after drinking. You must be ready to face these aspects of yourself head on to finally be relieved of the hold they have on you. When you confront the frightening aspects of yourself, they can be released fully, making you feel lighter and freer after the ceremony is complete.

This is going to be the most taxing journey you have most likely taken in your life. You must be forgiving and understanding with yourself. We all make mistakes and it is not the end of the world. Once you acknowledge these aspects, Madre Ayahuasca will release you from these situations as you have learned from them.

You may see people in your current life or those who are passed interspersed with alien or fairytale like creatures or animals. It is important to see the symbolism behind any visions you may have as they contain so much knowledge from Mother Ayahuasca to show you the way.

During this state is when you will feel that all energy, all beings, all creatures are one flowing mass which complement each other. There is no separation, judgement or authority. We are all equal in this state with ourselves and the environment around us.

You may experience an initial calm after all of the mayhem from you all your senses being pushed to their limits and then subsequently be pushed even higher into your consciousness to travel to other unimaginable dimensions. You may see divine beings, creatures, Mother Aya herself or even the devil or demons. The spiritual world comprises of everything good and evil. It is not your choice as to what is seen. You are shown what you need to see about yourself.

It is this higher state of consciousness that you will be able to answer the most common questions all human beings have of our purpose here on earth, whether God exists and how to move forward with this knowledge that you have uncovered within yourself. In this state, it will be rather difficult to relay your experiences as they are indescribable in words.

The clarity that is found for the unending patterns that seemingly cannot be broken is astonishing because of the objective view that you process while in communication with Mother Ayahuasca.

If you encounter visions during the ceremony, they may be coupled with distortions of sounds, audible hallucinations and noise you can visualize. As you can see, Aya takes you into an unimaginable space in which to work with her. In this frame of mind, you will be able to embrace this magical world of the paranormal. You will get lost in this world and lose all sense of time as we know it.

When the medicine is circling throughout every cell in your body, you will become more perceptive to all your senses. Everything from the smell of the incense, the environment around you and the sounds the participants are making will be greatly enhanced. This can cause a myriad of emotions to wash over you and bounce back between feeling an overwhelming amount of love and appreciation to getting highly agitated and irritated by the overstimulation.

When you accept that there is a whole range of possibilities that may occur with your ayahuasca experience, you will have a must deeper profound encounter with Mother Ayahuasca.

The visualizations start off slowly while coming over you in waves to crescendo into much stronger and enlightening visions. The longer you are able to see the visions, the more puzzling they may become and they heavily are based on symbolism.

Nobody can tell you what you will see in this hyper-dimensional plane. Anything goes and no rules apply. From spirits of the animals and safe worlds that the shaman creates with his sacred songs to mythical beings, demons, spirits, demi-gods, structures, ineffable sources of energy. Every experience is unique and none can be portrayed faithfully enough for you to get a picture of what it looks like. It's like being in a lucid dream of an alien.

With the mirror that Mother Ayahuasca puts in front of through your subconscious, you are simply faced with the truth of yourself and there is nowhere to hide when you are faced with the cold hard facts of who you truly are. So if there is something that you have been doing wrong with your life, Aya will show these things to you with an all knowing motherly smile on her face realizing it is something that you need to consciously be aware of for your overall betterment. There also is no way to unsee what you have seen, and, again, it is up to you to take the first step to remedying these wrongs and to start living your life in a more positive light.

Your body may take on different shapes or you may see that it is not a solid mass at all but rather blends into the energy of everything surrounding you.

Yawning is another way to release negative blockages in your body.

These negative aspects cover an array of emotional release such as hatred, regrets, fears, anxieties and self-loathing.

Sometimes you get to experience yourself inside your mother's womb. You feel as if you are actually present in the amniotic fluid and feeling the contractions of her muscles as you are being rebirthed in a spiritual way. You may also see the grander picture of how your parents and others felt and acted in the situation giving you insight into instances you probably have never thought about.

During the memories of conversations that you have had, you may have insight to what you should have said to be more gentle, loving and understanding in your relationships.

At first, you may feel dizzy with the force of speed the colors and shapes that occur during the visionary stage.

Because of the profound realizations, the psychological effects may last for weeks as you dissect the meaning behind the symbolism on your lessons. It will take time and you must be forgiving, kind and understanding with yourself. Do not rush into any rash decisions that violate your intuition.

If you are dealing with feeling lost or a life threatening disease, you will likely visualize what is known as the void. This is a space which is infinite and completely black nothingness. It has been thought this place is death itself as nothing seems to exist in this space, but it is the Ultimate herself. You can face your deepest fears within this space and be cradled by Her. If you find yourself in this space, be certain to be in a surrendering attitude, and your spiritual aspects will soar in ways you never thought possible. This is a precious gift and is not to be feared.

This is also the attitude that you need to maintain throughout the entire ceremony. Of course it is natural to feel fear when you take your first drink because fear is based on what you do not know. Once you have an understanding of the worlds you are going to encounter, that fear will dissipate when you focus on your intention and continue the process of surrender. Trust that the Shaman has created this safe space for you to face yourself and that no harm will come to you.

With this said, there are absolutely no limits other than your own thought process that will keep you from reaching the highest highs. This does not mean you will not experience any lows. But remember that you must go through the darkness to fully appreciate the light.

In the scientific studies related to the full five sense effects of drinking ayahuasca, they found the higher the dose of DMT, the more intense the visuals became. The visuals were not present the entire time and came in increments coupled with the physical purging. The visuals that were encountered were patterns that would move rather quickly, vibrations that were present in the visual field and absolute clarity of objects observed as if magnified. This was the case whether the subject's eyes were open or closed. They reported feeling as if they were in a dream state yet conscious of all that was happening in and around them.

The sounds the subjects heard were much more distinct and loud as if in a cave.

The rate of cognitive processes was greatly enhanced in a focused fashion helping them to take in the massive amounts of personal memories and information being presented on a psychological level. Much like watching a movie in fast forward but having complete understanding of what was occurring.

The emotions that were being recorded were extremely intense and included a range from amazement and utter sadness. There were also instances these emotions were simultaneously expressed.

There were also reports of leaving the body as well as an overwhelming euphoric feeling for others and the Universe.

As for the diet, there are many people who claim they have not had any ill effects from not following the recommendations. Overall it has been found that when you make your body as clean as possible, the effects of the ayahuasca are significantly more profound. This is due to you communing with the highest deity spirit and purity is the plane in which she works best. This is why the purging needs to take place.

If you did not take the advice of the all-important diet or *la dieta* prior to drinking, the Master plant will make sure to purify your body so that it can do the greatest work. If you followed the diet ahead of time as recommended by your specific Shaman, the Spirit will be able to communicate with you on a deeper level and you will have a more profound experience.

You must also think that the Shamans have been following this diet for the whole of their lives, especially while learning about and using Ayahuasca. Westerners are accustomed to their specific diet and these impurities have been building up over an entire lifetime. So even if you follow the Amazonian diet as prescribed for a short period of time, you will most likely not avoid the common effect of purging or *la purge* during the ceremony.

This is not a reaction to the medicine that you should shun, however. This is seen as a release of all the negativity that has been blocking energy from correctly flowing through your subtle energy body as well as your physical body. It is the reason for illness and disease and should be a welcome aspect. This does not make the act of purging any less intense. The most common method of purging is through vomiting or defecating but can also be released through tears, laughter or a combination. The key is to keep the correct mindset and your thoughts on your intention of what you brought you there in the first place to know that all of this is for your greater good.

Even people who do not normally cry or laugh may have this reaction during the purging process.

It has been documented that while being in this diminished physical state which also is accompanied with challenging alterations in your consciousness that you may end up unconsciously harming others or yourself. This is where the facilitators come into the ceremony as they assist the Shaman in looking for the warning signs and come to help you re-center. A true Shaman will stay for the entire event and not leave the facilitators and participants to fend for themselves.

After the ceremony, you will find your energy levels will skyrocket and that you will have less fear. You may change your entire life or small aspects that will hugely impact your daily life. It may change your ideals and beliefs. Anything is possible when it comes to ayahuasca because you are tapping into infinite wisdom.

As time passes, you will slowly come down from the Master plant and be in a state of peace and joyousness. You will likely be tired after this emotional and physical ordeal but your mind will be aware and clear.

Usually if you spend time at an extended retreat center, you are going to feel your emotions and body go through a proverbial roller coaster. This is where it is helpful to experience ayahuasca through a center as there are usually facilitators that are available throughout the day for you to talk through what you are going through.

You will find many people will create paintings or songs about these type of experience as it is the only way to somewhat grasp what was seen.

These effects can last for days, even weeks, after the ceremony. You would be living the term *high on life* and feel more empathy for the environment and people you encounter.

Because you will be experiencing heightened levels of energy, you will feel determined to implement the lessons that were taught during the session, sometimes rearranging your entire life. Not every person's experience is that extreme, but you get out what you put into your personal Ayahuasca communion.

You will find that the experience may even change your eating habits by shying away from unhealthy choices and you will keep your distance from negative events, people and thoughts that could bring harm to you emotionally.

When there is a friendly and nurturing environment surrounding the entire journey, it brings the group closer together to be able to process the encounters that Madre Aya gifts as well as to integrate those lessons in a safe atmosphere.

If you fail to fully integrate the lessons that were learned through Mother Aya, you will cycle back to the way you were before and have an interesting story to tell to those who are interested. You will likely forget the profound epiphanies that you encountered. It is hard to believe that after going through such an awkward exchange between your ego and Mother Ayahuasca to have this come to pass. However, it is a very real outcome. Do not let this opportunity to achieve the reasons which brought you to commune with Spirit herself go in vain.

No matter the results of your night with Aya – whether you experienced the highest highs or the darkest lows, you will get exactly what you need. The definition of positive and negative is a concept that needs a fresh perspective as the result will always be a better version of you if you allow it to be by integrating your lessons.

Even though ayahuasca is an entheogenic, the trip that you receive cannot be compared to mushrooms or LSD encounters you may have experienced.

Do not feel discouraged if you felt like you lost an opportunity to communicate with the visions that you encountered. If you are in a retreat center, you are likely going to be having several ceremonies within a selected period of time. Sometimes there are additional sessions that you can participate in if you feel like you need to dig deeper into your journey.

If you chose to go through more sessions with Madre Ayahuasca, you will find that you have become more familiar with the process and you will be able to focus your intention more deeply to gain answers to specific questions. There will be more clarity in the visuals and symbols that you see during the ceremony and will therefore be able to integrate the lessons easily.

The Sexual Aspect

With sex being such a grand part of the Western lifestyle, it be quite confusing to some of why the preparations for the ceremonies specifically say to refrain from having sex or even masturbating for at least two weeks before and at least a week after the ceremony. For some people, this would feel like a privacy of their inner freedom to enjoy this side of their life. However, there is a deeper meaning as to why this is prescribed.

Sexual energy is the most potent energy that can be created within your body. When you start to work with it in a focused and meaningful way, it can be the catalyst to opening up your spiritual connection to the Divine. Because the master plant spirits operate in a much higher frequency vibration, the preparation tools that the Shamans prescribe are meant to bring your body at the highest frequency that it can be. It would be a matter of trying to meet the spirits half way so to speak. The less dense you are by following the diet and sexual protocol, the easier it will be for the spirits of the master plants to be able to communicate with you.

This would, in theory, also minimize the amount of purging that would need to occur because the sexual energy known as kundalini or Shakti are known to be extremely healing and will clear these pathways for you while it builds up in your system.

It is also because the spirits of the master plants get very jealous when sexual energy is wasted on human beings rather than placing that energy towards connecting them. Because they are very sensitive to energies, the master plant spirits are able to sense the sexual energy when released into the subtle body energy. This is turn creates a dense factor in your aura that goes against the vibration they work from.

When you have your sexual energy flowing through your chakras as it is meant to, your sexual energy or Kundalini will rise through the chakras and open the third eye when the pineal gland is activated through the DMT. This will then leave you as an open channel to receive the teachings that Mother Aya has to offer without impediment.

When your sexual energy has been depleted through sex or masturbation, your energy levels need time to rebuild once again to peak levels. This usually takes a conscious effort and takes at least a week to get to the higher levels without concentration on the effort. With the kundalini levels being lowered, it will be more difficult to reach a higher vibration to be able to commune with Mother Ayahuasca.

When you are dealing with the master plants, purity is key. When you have sexual relations with others, your energy is tainted with the other person's energy. Where this is not necessarily a bad thing in our world, this makes it rather difficult for the master plant to be able to do her work as she perceives it as a tainted, impure environment to work in.

Refraining from orgasming will also keep your energy levels sexually and physically at their peak and allow you to have the strength and stamina needed to get through the ceremony while learning everything that Madre Aya has to show.

If you think that it is worth masturbating or having sex while giving up your chance to have actual healing performed on your body, maybe you should take a step back to reevaluate your priorities when it comes to having the ayahuasca experience. Just like you are going to need to work personally towards healing yourself through the wisdom that Mother Ayahuasca bestows, this is showing her as well that you are willing to sacrifice something that she knows is important to Westerners to receive her grace.

It is also a matter of respect to Mother Aya as well as to your commitment to your Shaman that you agreed to. If you are not willing to follow and respect your agreements that you swore to, then, again, your intentions need to have a serious look over.

The benefits will far outweigh what you are giving up. You will find that conserving your sexual energy and Shakti will actually aid you in ways you probably are not aware of.

When you look at Eastern religions, the holy men and women abstain from sexual intercourse during their quest for attaining enlightenment. You see this across many religions and cultures with similar backgrounds to the indigenous people of the Amazon Basin. When you put what they are asking you do in their perspective and context, there is a viable reason why they are asking you to perform these specific preparations. Otherwise, they would not have mentioned anything about the subject.

If you are interested in harnessing your sexual energy to the highest levels for the ceremony, you can research tantric practices to raise your kundalini levels. You can also ask your shaman about the ways they suggest you do this to prepare you properly for the ceremony.

Some easy techniques to getting in touch with your kundalini are to focus on your heart chakra while taking in deep breaths. Take note of the subtle body energy that surrounds you as you continue to take deep breaths. Connect with this energy and start to consciously breathe it in, pushing it to anywhere in your body that feels like there is a blockage or tightness. Shakti will start to heal those areas and break the blockages down to dissipate them fully.

Another technique is to focus on the base of your back where your spine is located. Connect with your subtle body energy again by sensing the Shakti flowing from the base of your spine up to the top of your head where the crown chakra is located. Then lower the energy back down to the heart chakra and continue to breathe the subtle body energy. Then again lower the Shakti with your breath back down to the bottom of your spine.

The second rotation would go only up to your heart chakra. Feel how the energy is clearing out your meridians and chakras. Breathe the energy into your body and then push it down again to your spine.

If you perform these exercises during the days that you are to be abstinent, this will build your sexual energy to its peak and you will certainly have a higher vibration. This again will facilitate the communion with Mother Ayahuasca, and you will be more clear and open for whatever she would like for you to experience.

Redefining Your Ego as You Know It

When one looks at the aspects of the mind, body and spirit being interconnected, it can easily be believed that the ego is the basis for much of the imbalance that is experienced in the body. Since the ego is based in fear, this can crop up in nasty physical ways be in cancer or an autoimmune disorder. If your ego is of the angry type, you can have cardiovascular, blood pressure issues as well as depression as a symptom of your egos response to feeling assaulted. As this feeling of assault continues, the downward spiral of detaching yourself from your normal social engagements or even finding pleasure in the hobbies you used to enjoy is stripped away. All because of a bruised and angry ego.

Think of your ego as an actor. The best perceived version you have of yourself and who you present out to the people in the world. It is the opposite of your authentic self. When you drink the ayahuasca brew, this is the greatest injustice that you could serve to your ego - from the ego's perspective. There is no way for ego to survive in the world of authenticity, especially being the case in the world of Mother Aya.

In this world, you are reminded that you can harness a deep inner strength that was present all along whereas your ego may make you feel incapable of achieving the life you always dreamed of.

Know one thing - once you drink ayahuasca, there is no going back during the ceremony or ever to be the person you were before you took that drink. For some, this is a welcome aspect. For most, this is frightening. But considering some of the reasons that people come to the ceremony to seek true change or healing, they are the ones who take the most away from the experience itself.

The reason that many people fail to see improvement while relying on psychotherapy to solve their problems is that it fully reinforces the ego defenses. All the issues that are supposedly being faced head on is just a manifestation of the identification of the ego and it preserving itself at all costs. On the other hand, when ayahuasca is used to receive help with your problems, the walls of the ego are removed as they cannot exist in the world with Mother Aya.

She allows you to see yourself with the full slate of information and with a new perspective. It is like you are sitting on a speeding train looking out the window as the information comes to you at light speed. It is hard to take it all in at the time or even in the "right" time as time is an illusion in her world. The integration period will help you to be able to put the puzzle pieces together in a linear fashion that your brain can understand. You will have continuing epiphanies as long as you stay in that space with her, continuing to be open to what she still has to teach you. It is a conscious effort that you probably will not get correct the first time as you usually need support to be guided in the right directions so as to not lose your footing.

When you slip out of her world, you unconsciously step back into your old patterns and way of living life. You will not notice this until you have lost the connection.

Through the meeting of Madre Aya, you are given the gift of a richer and more enhanced life full of joy. You can let things slide off your back as you realize they hold no importance. You can feel like yourself and love yourself more. You will likely have more generosity and humility while realizing there is an important aspect in love that has been lacking in your life. It will flip your perspective on everything, if you allow her to do her work and not step in the way with your ego and expectations.

To get past the door, you must leave your ego at the door. There is no go forward with that baggage on your shoulder. And there is no going back to the person you defined yourself to be once you do.

The ego has been allowed to be reinforced by repeated patterns which has it revealing it its own statute and false glory. It believes that it has a place in all the unfolding drama in your life that it borders on the state of arrogance. With ego being constantly fed by you playing into your feelings of fear and acting the role of the victim, it becomes a ravenous animal which consumes you unknowingly.

may find the results of ayahuasca to further disintegrate their ego strength, causing increased disorganization and confused boundaries.

When the wisdom of Mother Ayahuasca shines the light on your ego, the boundaries that once were set are faded and leaves you in a state of feeling like you are losing your mind. The identity that you have aided in creating is being forced to show its true colors of falsehood. The façade is seen plain as day and cannot be denied by any person who knows what is best for their consciousness. The truth of the intentions of ego to continue to grasp onto control by repressing these traumas and imprints of difficult situations you have been through is finally revealed.

This is the most difficult part of the process for most as this can feel like the ultimate stab in the back, and you were the one that was doing it to yourself the entire time. Bringing back the insights of this realization is the most beneficial to your integration process and shifting your life to live more authentically.

The Process of Dissolution & Death of the Ego

The instinct of our egos is to hide and run away from these realizations instead of facing them head on. This is the wrong intention to have during an ayahuasca ceremony as you are resisting the very core of the lessons you were brought there to learn. This perspective also can bring you into the more negative and darker aspects of your ego if you chose it over the all-powerful and knowing Spirit of the Vine. Surrender to Aya by accepting your vulnerability and letting go to the entire experience, and it will likely take you to greater heights physically, mentally and spiritually.

When you realize that you are not the one in control of yourself to include your reactions, feelings and thoughts or even that you know yourself better than this Master plant is when you start to go through the painful yet beautiful process of the death of your ego. This occurs when you are completely trusting of the knowledge that Madre Aya gives to you and you see yourself and everything she is teaching you at face value.

As for the negative aspects you may encounter, fear will be the most common because this is the tool of your ego. Because of your ego going through a traumatic state, you may be flooded with feelings of losing your mind, paranoia and feeling as if you are dying. This in fact is the process of the ego death and can be a life altering spiritual revelation. This is due mainly in part of realizing and reliving past memories and traumas.

Even after experiencing an ego death, it is rather difficult to maintain this belief when you position yourself back into your old life and the world that you knew before the ceremony. This is the reason why many people decide to turn their lives upside down in an effort to stay true to their authentic selves.

Ego Death is a process that can be a temporary or full immersion into the death of how you define yourself within the concepts of this world. This can be defined in several different ways depending on religious and cultural background, education, age, personal experiences with prior altered states of consciousness. It is where you conceive yourself in a different perspective that your pre-conceptualized version of yourself.

The main effect that people feel when going through this process is that they do not see themselves separate from other people or the environment. It is not all about you anymore as you realize that there is no singular you. Being of the same energy and essence of everything in the world, you are no longer trying to be a distinct entity or separate from what you are naturally a part of.

This idea is seen in many eastern religions where the goal is to transcend the attachments of this world while on the path to awakening and enlightenment. It can also be described as being in the state of having no mind as you realize that the thoughts that are created in your head are not your own.

During this process you lose the barrier between the objective world and what you have conceived as yourself. You then will have the sense of oneness with the entire Universe and every person and object contained within. This is usually coupled with a visual display of a bright golden or white light or a range of colors like the rainbow.

Using ayahuasca to achieve ego dissolution is usually a temporary measure. However, it gives you the faith that these other planes exist and as such will alter reality as you know it currently. While going through the dying of the ego, you feel as if you are losing yourself because everything that you defined as being "you" is an illusion. It is a concept that you have created to be able to live in the constructs of this world. You will find if you continue down this path that you will find who you truly are after losing this identity that you have created.

This is a sign of spiritual awakening through the use of ayahuasca and is a very heightened way of experiencing the medicine. It is during this process that you will gain the most insight into who you have created yourself to be compared to who you truly are.

CHAPTER 4

Ayahuasca's Healing Powers

There are many facets of healing that the ayahuasca brew has been bringing to the table for thousands of years. Since the knowledge of this medicine has been spreading for the last forty years, the use has expanded from being a divining and healing tool used by the local shamans. The spiritual awakenings that have been reported while using this master plant has grown since being popularized into the Aya ceremonies that we know today.

As with all sacred plants, it needs to be respected and not overused. Long term use is sometimes prescribed while using the method of micro dosing for those who suffer from significant mental and physical issues. However, some patients who have chronic illnesses realize significant alterations in their health only after three ceremonies that have commenced during a short period of time.

Too much of a good thing is true when it comes to drinking ayahuasca as Westerners are able to overdose on this substance. The short term effects that can be experienced are muscle spasms, dizziness, vertigo, sedation, motor function impairment, sweating, hyperthermia, autonomic instability and tremors. After scientific study, it has been determined these effects are caused by the harmala alkaloids that are present in the ayahuasca vine.

As stated before, everyone has a different outcome when taking Aya. Some people may not see the benefits after drinking which may lead them to abusing the medicine to get the expected resolution to their issues. Due to the high concentrations of serotonin in the brew, it is best not to use more than what you require. When you have an overdose, this could lead to what is known as serotonin syndrome which will have a much more negative effect such as dark flashbacks and prolonged trips. If you follow the guidelines on how to properly use ayahuasca for your greatest benefit, this will not be the outcome.

The hallucinogenic effects of the brew cannot be compared to other entheogenic substances such as mushrooms or LSD. Instead of losing yourself in the experience, you will find that you have a heightened sense of awareness of everything that is occurring around you.

When you witness the seemingly impossible worlds through the use of ayahuasca, you can come to believe that anything is possible. With this belief system being solidified, you are able to face anything without fear and thus are more free physically, mentally and spiritually.

With so many personal accounts coming to light of treatment and healings being conducted using the ayahuasca brew, there are many interested scientists who are wanting to understand the scientific side of this healing plant combination. Of course this curiosity helps the scientists to be creative in how these studies are being conducted. The more popular the master plant becomes, the more demand for these types of studies will be conducted. For those that are more spiritually minded people, they do not need the proof of science to know that drinking ayahuasca works to heal the body on all levels.

With DMT being an illegal drug for much of the world, it is rather difficult to be able to test each component. Different branches of retreat centers and churches have been able to incorporate the use of ayahuasca brew for the most part without being disturbed due to the religious basis of the ceremonies.

Now the studies are digging deeper to find out if ayahuasca is effective for treating other disorders and diseases. Knowing that the mind, body and spirit are interconnected, it could be said that a whole range of illnesses can be treated while using the brew. However, some people need the science to back these claims up as they would need to be dependent on pharmaceutical medications otherwise.

When these scientists have an open and aware mind while researching these plants, they will realize overall that nature is better and more knowledgeable doctors to treat the patient's bodies than modern science in some instances.

If you should go to Brazil for the ceremony, they have integrated the Santo Daime Church and UDV belief systems with the frequent use of the Ayahuasca tea. It has been found that members participate in a ceremony once weekly and have lesser occurrences of mental health and addiction issues as a whole.

The General Benefits

Creativity being strengthened is another benefit of drinking the tea as it puts you more in touch with these aspects of yourself. Because you are more aware of the world around you, everything potentially is an avenue for inspiration and it brings inner focus which makes you more productive on any projects you may be working on in the workplace as well as your personal life.

You may find that your creative side gets more colorful and innovative as your mind will be more clear to focus on new ideas. This can also be the case in any aspect of your life. This is also coupled with your new sense of heightened energy levels which will help you to accomplish any goal you set for yourself.

Because of the revelations that are realized after drinking Aya, you will find that you are more relaxed and happier. Studies have shown the connection between overall gratefulness and happiness to correlate directly to the higher level of health found in these individuals. This also strengthens the idea that your thoughts heavily influence your outer world. When you are in this state of mind, you will naturally keep elevating the cycle while connecting to higher vibrations while you awaken to your full potential.

Fear has less of a hold on your life as you are able to easily take leaps of faith that you would have been reluctant to exercise before the ceremony. These instances are usually positive shifts for the individual which aid them in living their life to their full potential and highest purpose.

The ego is the basis for fear and the ayahuasca experience has a way of shattering or eliminating the ego altogether. As such, when ego is less in the picture, you are free to live your life without fear. This has a noticeable impact for those who suffer from debilitating fear based illnesses as it affects them across the board mentally, spiritually and physically. This is due to the interconnection of the mental, spiritual and physical aspects, when you deal with one aspect, the others in turn are affected.

When Mother Aya shows you exactly what you have been hiding from yourself, you will find the path of acceptance and integration of the lessons will have the highest benefit for you with all aspects of yourself. This experience can bring psychological and physical distress. However, if you see this as an amazing opportunity to let go of the things that are holding you back in life, you will see the greatest impact on your life. If you have the perspective that all happens is for your greater good, you will look upon the negative experiences in a higher perspective. Not everything worth gaining is easy, and this is especially true when taking this intention in with you to the ceremony.

The medicine gives you the insight and you must choose how to use that information to move forward in a more positive manner.

This link between the physical, mental and spiritual aspects have been studied. The results concluded that when a person had gone through an emotional trauma during their lives, especially during childhood, it directly correlated to having a higher risk of developing liver disease, skeletal fractures, lung disease, cardiovascular disease and cancer. It also was found that the spiritual aspect was lacking or non-existent.

When you work properly with the Spirit of the Vine, you are able to be freed from the effects of the trauma that you have experienced. In effect, it recalibrated the balance between the physical, mental and spiritual aspects, resulting in a happier and healthier being after drinking Aya.

Results from drinking the brew showed a range of outcomes which were based on being more aware of nature and relationships with the people. There was an understanding of how all these aspects are interconnected and created a sense of empathy, love and compassion for the universe and everything contained within.

You realize that every living creature has a spirit and you feel the interconnectedness with everything in the universe. Through this process, you will see a breakdown or dissolution of the ego. You may even experience the loss of your ego completely.

This spiritual awakening has a noticeable impact on how you live your life after the ayahuasca journey. Through the knowledge that you gain, you will continue to encounter deep revelations, continued spiritual awakening encounters as well as a full understanding of your purpose in this world. The journey never has to end as ayahuasca opens a doorway into your inner consciousness which contains an infinite amount of knowledge.

One of the main uses that the ayahuasca vine was used for in the indigenous communities was to eliminate parasites within the body. This was a physical aspect of the act of purging. This coupled up with the spiritual cleansing process to remove any negative aspects.

With more scientific studies substantiating the benefits of ayahuasca, it still may be difficult to grasp these seemingly far out concepts. However, if you are put in the position in your life where you are completely stuck or faced with a life debilitating situation where you see no way forward, this is the opportunity to take a leap of faith into the unknown. If nothing else has been working for you to get out of this mind set, you need to simply trust that you may not have all of the answers and turn off your analytical, rational mind to think outside of the box. You may be surprised by what you discover.

Scientists are also looking outside of the analytical box to find that there is supporting evidence that transpersonal encounters are important to psychological health and overall wellbeing. Because ayahuasca use leads to marked improvements in behavior and psychological changes, it is one of the best avenues to consider when needing therapeutic assistance.

Post-Traumatic Stress Disorder

In respect of PTSD, is has been found that drinking ayahuasca will help you to come to terms with the traumas that center around this disease. It will help you to become more honest with the real reasons why you are reacting the way that you are to everyday situations. Then you are able to retrain your brain with your new perspective on life and reverse reactions you have to the outside stimuli. Using this method, it treats this disease more effectively than pharmaceutical means which cover up the basis of the creation of PTSD. It has shown that even the side of effects of suicidal thoughts are cleared from the mind after drinking ayahuasca.

When sufferers of PTSD go through the awakening process that ayahuasca provides, they usually witness the traumatic experiences in which their illness stems. This time, they relive the moments but without the intense emotions they have associated with these recurring memories. They are also able to utilize the object view that comes with the ayahuasca experience to be able to see the bigger picture of the trauma they encountered.

Overall, ayahuasca transforms your spirit and mind to be cleared and reconditioned. When this occurs, you realize the healing and health benefits associated with living in that state of awareness.

Eating Disorders

With the advent of the scientific research being conducted, they are starting to look to other disorders that can possibly be treated or cured through the use of ayahuasca tea. Eating disorders are on this list and starting to see some results.

There are studies ongoing showing that the serotonin function abnormalities are the cause of many dysfunctions in thought process which lead to eating disorders.

When DMT is introduced to remedy the low levels of serotonin, this neurotransmission is able to bind to the 2A receptors of the brain. This leads to a calmer thought process treating the root of the problem.

Depression and Anxiety

In a particular study about the effects of ayahuasca brew in regards to chronic depression, there were promising results backed by science about this ancient medicine plant.

There were two study groups in a particular study. One was given ayahuasca as the other was given a placebo. The day after the study began, a depression test was conducted. The ayahuasca group had the highest scores compared to the placebo group. The same test was conducted after seven days with different results. The placebo group had dropped back down to their depression levels at the beginning of the study whereas the ayahuasca group had continued to raise their scores higher than before. It was concluded that Aya was capable of decreasing the effects of depression and increasing an overall sense of spirituality.

It has been further proven through other scientific studies that depression is greatly reduced within three hours after drinking the medicine. Due to the similarities of the master plant to pharmaceutical antidepressants, it acts in the same way by altering the concentration of serotonin in the brain. However, with the added component of DMT within the brew, it adds in the necessary spiritual aspect to fully treat the illness. Facing your fears and traumas head on is directly correlated to the impact that the Aya brew has on depression. You must have the determination and courage to be able to resolve the issues to finally be relieved of your physical symptoms.

Cancer

There have been countless reports of people with serious life threatening cancers being completely cured. The active ingredient of the harmine found in the ayahuasca is responsible for the cell structures to be altered, reversing the cancer cell structure completely.

Addictions

It has been studied how ayahuasca brew can reduce or eradicate dependencies and addictions. The science behind addictions such as smoking, alcohol or other recreational drugs are due to a serotonin deficiency. Because the brew of ayahuasca has a high concentration of serotonin, this brings the serotonin levels back to a normal level. This then decreases the cravings for said drug which leads to you no longer relying on the drug for the serotonin input.

Mental Health Disorders

It is wise to refrain from drinking ayahuasca brew if you have a history with mental illness, even if it has been dormant. This may result in a psychotic episode. On rare occasions, this has also come to pass with mentally healthy people. Be sure to have a person that the retreat center or ceremony facilitator can contact if necessary.

If you are someone who suffers from bipolar disorder, personality disorders, psychosis or schizophrenia, you are a higher risk admission into a ceremony. This does not mean you will not be taken at all. However, the chances of acceptance are slimmer when the psychiatric disorder is currently active. Honesty is the best policy when it comes to informing potential retreat centers and shamans so that everyone is on the same page as to what is being dealt with.

Even though it is understood that pharmaceutical medications and therapies are not always ideal, this does not mean that all alternative and natural therapies are right for every person.

There have been success stories when it comes to people with a history of mental disorders. However, there have been instances in which the partaker's symptoms came back. Be sure you have the support and sincerity of a safe space in which to facilitate healing for you and know that you are going to be taken care of given any situation.

There have been marked health differences in people with mental health disorders implementing more spiritual measures in their life including prayer, yoga and meditation. This is turn makes the patient more aware of their body's needs and an overall feeling of connectedness and awareness to their bodies.

Overall Health Benefits

In recent years, there has been increased interest in the effect that ayahuasca has on the treatment and cures for difficult to treat ailments of addiction, cancer, post-traumatic stress disorder (PTSD), eating disorders and depression. There has been an array of biomedical studies on the matter.

There have been instances where supposedly incurable diseases have been treated through the use of ayahuasca. When it comes to things of this nature occurring, one's mind may go straight to the thought of it being a miracle or a gift from God. On one hand it may be just that. However, your body has an amazing capacity to heal if given the opportunity. It is a matter of a balance. For your body to be in a healthy state, your mind must be in balance which also correlates to the spiritual aspect of our beings. When they all align, you will find that illness and petty things like worry and anxiety will not impact you so negatively.

The illness that it felt in the body is due to an emotional trauma that is still being clutched onto. Many times this event is so painful that it is locked away in the confines of your subconscious to be seemingly forgotten. However, through the use of the ayahuasca brew, these memories come through as if they happened yesterday so that they can finally be dealt with. Once they are, the hold these situations had on you will be released. This results in feeling the effects of this release rather quickly if not instantly and will last as long as there are no traumas left to release. You may find that you have a temporary relief from pain or mental issues, and this would mean that you have to dig deeper into the reason why these are happening.

Illness that occur in your body are major teachers for lessons that must be learned in this life. If you have not learned the lesson, these ailments will continue to be present until they are dealt with directly. Using the medicine of ayahuasca greatly assists in this process and is why many people are turning to this ancient brew for direction as they may have exhausted all other medical treatments and options.

The total process beginning with the cleansing of your body through the experience of Aya herself and integrating what was realized results in a reset of the default activity in the brain. In other words, you break old patterns which automatically tell your brain to feel certain pain. This has proven to be an effective tool to neutralize emotional pain which exhibits itself through physical symptoms experienced in the body.

Depending on the amount of past traumas that are directly dealt with, this will correlate to how long the symptoms will subside. This is why people with more chronic symptoms need to have a longer healing period using ayahuasca on multiple occasions to dig deep enough to address all psychological issues.

This master plant even affects the immune system through the T cells. Because these T cells have receptors for serotonin, after drinking the brew you will notice a reduction of inflammation throughout the body within a couple of hours.

Health Risks with Ayahuasca Tea & Pharmaceutical Medicine

When using the extremely powerful master plant of ayahuasca, you must realize the negative effects that traditional medicine has on this plant medicine working correctly. It can have major health implications when you mix the two. Having less in your system is best when it comes to utilizing the healing power of ayahuasca. The biggest culprit for fatal reactions are selective serotonin reuptake inhibitor (SSRI) medications. Studies directly with DMT have been carried out to realize the medical benefits of the main hallucinogenic component of Aya tea. They found that when the effects were at their peak at approximately the 2-hour mark, this is when the DMT was found to be in the greatest quantity in the blood.

After seventy-five minutes, the diastolic blood pressure readings significantly rose 9 mm Hg for the higher doses of DMT. They noticed that the heart rate and systolic blood pressure was very slightly increased during the study.

The other heavy hitter that you do not want to combine with ayahuasca brew is MAOIs. If you do combine these medications with Aya, they can cause unwanted results of cerebrovascular disease, cardiovascular disease, hypertension, severe headaches as well as severe kidney and liver impairment.

When imbalances are felt through all aspects of the body, it is a sign that you are comfortable within yourself and not living your life authentically. When it comes to treating illnesses, you need to have a candid conversation with your doctor. Even if you think they will not be open to the idea of you using master plants for healing, it is best to get their advice. You also have the right to seek a second opinion if you feel like you are not getting all the answers that you require.

Medical conditions that need special attention during ayahuasca ceremonies are pregnancy, diabetes, liver and kidney conditions, epilepsy, cardiovascular ailments, psychosis, bipolar syndrome and schizophrenia.

Conditions that will get you automatically declined to sit at a ceremony are cardiovascular illnesses and high blood pressure as the DMT contained in the brew raises your blood pressure to higher than normal levels. Bipolar disorder is also a tricky mental illness as the effects could easily cause a manic episode, potentially putting the other participants at risk.

If you are experiencing other medical syndromes, talk directly with the facilitator or Shaman if able to determine the best master plants to use for you personally. Keep in mind, not all Shamans are qualified to handle these extreme health ailments, and some may turn you away. Do not get discouraged because there are fully trained Shamans who are willing to help those suffering from chronic diseases.

Spiritual Benefits

There are also many reports of people feeling as if they have gone through the process of death only to be reborn again. It helped to locate the connection that they felt they had lost and made them remember that all life is sacred.

A particular study showed that long term users of ayahuasca as a spiritual tool score high in all nine aspects of the Spiritual Orientation Inventory. The nine categories include fruits of spirituality, awareness of the tragic, idealism, altruism, material values, sacredness of life, mission in life, purpose in life, meaning of life and transcendent dimension.

Using ayahuasca is like putting the puzzle pieces of your life together in a way that you can clearly understand. You are shown your behaviors and reactions in your conscious and unconscious mind and how they relate and affect your relationships. You see how these reactions are imprinted on you through outside sources and how to stop the cycle. Likewise, you may also experience a physical healing of your body as divine entities or Madre Aya working directly with you in a tangible way.

You may feel complete loneliness and fear as you are faced with the wisdom of the ways of the world and how you interconnect to everything. You can feel the connection to the spirits of nature, the food that you consume and the air that you breathe and how they all correlate with each other.

You may find along with a heightened sense of physical and mental energy that you possess that you will find that you do not need much food or sleep to keep the same energy levels. This is due to the fact that you are tapping into the internal energy within your subtle body and less connected to the world as you know it. This is a sign of spiritual awakening and you are on a long and hard path to enlightenment.

As it has been established, when there is a lack in one aspect of our mind, body and spirit, the imbalance will show up as an illness in one or more of those categories as they all correlate with each other. You can find the problems of anxiety and depression are closely related to a disconnect that we have with our higher self because of the society that we live in today. Instead of looking for higher planes, we are wondering which house we are going to buy or if our best friend is going to think we look fat in this dress.

We as a society are wholly consumed by what others think and how we are going to be judged. We waste so much energy and time worrying about petty things that only matter in this world. We could be using that energy to do so many better things in the world around us and within ourselves.

When you turn to ayahuasca to find deeper meaning to your life, you will likely walk away with your wish with gratitude and thankfulness for the gifts you have in your life. You will likely easily cut out people, places and things that no longer serve you that perhaps brought these negative aspects into your life. You will appreciate all the time that you have and share that time with others in a meaningful way.

In the words of Einstein, *No problem can be solved from the same level of consciousness that created it.* This shows that ayahuasca is a viable option in finding the solutions to your deep rooted baggage you have been dragging around with you for all these years.

You will find one you are able to drop that baggage, you will not only be free of the physical burden, but you will also be free to live more consciously wish takes far less effort than the life you are living now. When you live your life conscious and aware, you will notice the environment and people around you more. This will in turn have you feel more empathy to the joys and sufferings that are contained within this world. You will be more willing to help others and be less self-centered and selfish.

Anything that goes against your inner true self will naturally be revolting. This does not mean that you will be judgmental in its place. This means that your world will contain everything that you notice and are aware of. You will be able to see the instances that you can be more loving towards your family and friends. You will be able to pick up on others needing a helping hand or if something is off and they need a listening ear. You will become more present and attentive. Your life will take on a whole different meaning.

CHAPTER 5

How To Get The Most Out Of Your Journey With Ayahuasca

Choose Your Setting

When choosing a location, it is important to focus on what is your personal goals for this experience. Do you have the need to be with the indigenous tribes in the forests of the Amazon to get the true experience or do you think that you will need a bit more pampering after the event? Go after the ceremony that fits with your overall goal as there are faith based and traditional ceremonies to choose from. When you are in Brazil, the ritual of drinking Aya will likely be centered around the UVA and Santo Daime organizations. These ceremonies differ greatly from the traditional Amazonian rituals as they are based in Catholic roots. However, if this is your religion or you are Christian, it is worth incorporating your beliefs into the ceremony to make it that much more powerful for you.

While the usage of Aya is legal in Brazil and Peru, it is also legal in most places around the world as a religious right. So do not fret if you cannot leave your country to head to the Amazon directly. It will take a bit more diligence and asking the right people for direction, but again, Mother Ayahuasca will guide you to her when you are ready to see and listen.

If you are making sure that you are not being put into an awkward position, the Shamans in Ecuador are required to be certified and have paperwork to show to this effect. Be sure to inquire to ensure your Shaman has been properly trained to conduct the ceremony.

When you are vetting retreat centers, ensure that they have a system in place to analyze potential participants from attending. This is a method that should be in place to ensure people who could be potentially harmful to the overall benefits of the group are not admitted. They should also objectively inform you of any risks associated with drinking ayahuasca tea and screen you for your medical history.

They may even require you to have a doctor's note describing your health in detail before allowing you to reserve a session. If they start explaining that ayahuasca is a cure all or they promise you will have specific results after coming to their center, it is recommended to keep searching. Also, if the facilitator is not empathetic to your personal intentions and only boasting about how you have come to the best, it would be advised to find another center that deserves your trust.

Deal with the money issues before the ceremony. Be sure to have an understanding of what money is to be expected and what you should expect for the price you are paying. Also inquire as to when the money should be paid and to whom.

Find Peace

Before the ceremony, make sure that you calm your inner self by keeping a focus on meditation and breathing exercises that aid you in finding your center. Walk barefoot in the grass to ground yourself to the earth. Keep to yourself and silent to maintain your center. When you go into the ceremony, you are likely to have fear and anxiety about what is actually going to happen, but you must not let yourself be consumed by these feelings. If you do, you are likely to feel less of the medicinal effects or even nothing at all.

Keeping a sense of calm in knowing the fact that you are going to be faced with the truth and demons within yourself is no easy feat. Keeping your mind on lighter ideals and your intention will help you to break free of the battle of the ego that consumes us all.

Set a Heightened Awareness Intention

If you have concerns about it ayahuasca is something that you should do, highly consider taking a step back to reevaluate. What are your reasons for wanting to go through this journey?

Are you just wanting a life experience to brag to your friends about? Are you seeking for healing but have reservations about your state of health and if you can handle the medicine? Are you looking for a cure all for all your physical and psychological ailments? Are you wanting to gain the knowledge of how to better your relationships with the people around you and in the future? Are you feeling stuck in a whirlpool and do not know how to get out? You have tried other psychedelics and want to experience what this Master plant has to offer?

There are differing intentions that go through a person's mind before deciding to embark on this journey. Some are not the highest level of intentions that you can achieve and as such need to be reevaluated. If you are looking to ayahuasca to achieve an altered state of mind, to escape or for selfish reasons not in line with your higher self, it is best to look to other avenues. You must be in a higher state of mind when you embark on the journey with ayahuasca, or you may be in for a nasty ride. Because Spirit of the Vine is a powerful and knowledgeable medicine, it is best not to approach her with this attitude and mindset.

Take time to go into deep thought and contemplation about your intention behind doing this ceremony. It will be your anchor during the rough times of the process and be your celebrating point when the ceremony is complete. This will help you to keep your focus on the process as a whole as it can become quite distracting with so much going on at once. It should be completely personal to you, specific and something that you wholeheartedly believe in.

To give you some direction, are there any specific questions that you would like to learn from the Mother of the Universe? Do you have a specific problem within yourself that you are having difficulty finding a solution? Do you simply want to know who you can become? Also in the instance that find yourself having a conversation in the higher worlds with enlightened entities, it would be wise to take the opportunity to be able to get to the bottom of a few of your inquiries by tapping into that eternal knowledge.

Keeping focus on your intention also helps with this aspect and will dispel any fear or darkness that you may encounter. Be strong, brave and know that all these aspects are there to guide you in the right direction. Mother Ayahuasca knows what is best for you. If you do not have an amazing experience the first time, maybe it is because you did not let go, holding on fiercely to your ego and fear rather than trusting the Spirit. Maybe you were supposed to learn the ropes so the next time you drink, you will have a more profound experience. You will not have the insight into the methods of Madre Aya until after the ceremony is complete and perhaps not even for weeks afterwards.

Do not get upset if your intention or questions are not directly answered. The answers may show themselves in a later session or during your encounters with the world now that you have a different perspective on life.

Feel free to consult with your personal spiritual support you are already practicing to incorporate into the ceremony internally.

The Emotional Rollercoaster

If you are looking for a truly ego shattering life experience that you will keep with you each day to learn, grow and be more aware of the world and your place in it, then this is an avenue that you should consider. It is not an easy path or quick. With all things that are worth it, they take a great deal of dedication and perseverance to see it through to the end. Ayahuasca is not something that should be jumped into and takes preparation, time, humility and an open mind to gain the full benefit of the Spirits teachings.

Even with knowing what possibilities may occur for you after drinking the brew, ayahuasca does call out to people and draws them to her when they are ready. Just know that you are going to feel helpless and vulnerable while struggling with the truth of your subconscious.

Watch What You Consume

The dieta is a very important aspect of proper preparation and is quite different than the Western diet. You will need to incorporate raw and fresh vegetables and fruits which can easily be made from healthy juice combinations. However, be careful to avoid raspberries, pineapple, plums, raisins, figs, avocados and bananas.

You must refrain from eating pork & red meat, fried foods, caffeine, acidic foods, heavy spices, alcohol, processed foods, lentils, beans, peas, peanuts, dairy products, refined sugar and salt. This list also goes further into avoiding fermented foods, chocolate, fatty meals, protein extracts, foods which are pickled, soy & tamari sauce, sauerkraut, dried fruits and soy products. Some individuals perform a fast for a day or two prior to arriving to the retreat center or ceremony.

Depending on the beliefs of your Shaman, you may also get sacred mapacho tobacco cigarettes and Agua Florida to aid in purifies and cleansing the body during the ceremony.

Water is highly important as you will become dehydrated from the purging process and is a real danger if fluid levels are not kept up. Be sure to drink enough water in the days before the ceremony and also bring some water with you to the ritual itself. However, be sure not to overload yourself with water during the ceremony.

When you go through the recommendations of restrictions from Shamans beforehand, know that there are specific reasons why they are asking you to perform these actions. You need to be properly prepared for this intense experience and these recommendations will strengthen you spiritually and physically for the ceremony and in life in general. They give your circulatory and digestive system as well as your brain a much desired break and will cleanse them during the process.

For the experience of the ayahuasca journey energy to continue to reverberate through your body, keep the diet going for as long as possible after the ceremony. Not only will your body feel healthier, your energies will continue to skyrocket. You will find that this is not as cumbersome of a task as it may had been before the ceremony as you understand the purpose and reason behind ingesting healthy foods for your body.

No matter how much research you do on the subject of ayahuasca, there is no real way to be prepared for what you are getting yourself into. However, there are steps to prepare for your introduction to Mother Aya which will make it the best experience you can obtain.

If you are not able or willing to complete the entire scope of the diet, at the very least, ingest less salts and refined sugar for at least a couple of weeks. You can also keep your meals light and healthy and make sure that you are keeping a regimented exercise routine to prepare you physically for the experience.

Another facet of the diet is to make you more aware of the blockages that you are feeling as well as a way to connect to your body in a more conscious way. This is also a way to prepare yourself mentally, physically and spiritually for your ceremony encounter.

On the day of the ceremony, eat a small, light breakfast and have a high carbohydrate lunch. It is recommended to not eat at least 4 hours before your session and give yourself up to 6 hours if you have a slow metabolism.

Prepare Yourself Mentally for the Journey

The ceremony will push your boundaries to the utmost limit. This is the part that you simply cannot prepare for other than accepting this as fact. You are going to be faced with things within yourself that you have been ignoring or cannot face in your daily life. It will be a challenging endeavor. Humility of having the opportunity to partake in this Master plant will go a long way to helping you get through the rough patches where you just do not think that you can get through it. Keep calm and focused and, again, know that it will not last forever.

After you have drunk the ayahuasca, sit upright and wait for the medicine to reach every cell of your body. When you start to feel the effects of the Spirit, you can choose to lie down when you feel comfortable to do so. When the nausea hits, do not resist the medicine. Just surrender and allow the Spirit of the Vine to take you on the journey of a lifetime.

Try to go with the flow of things. You will have moments of nausea, moments where you will purge and others were you feel like you need to but nothing results. Do not expect anything of the process, be aware and be present in the moment by keeping your focus on your intention and breath. Everything will happen as it needs to if you just let Mother Ayahuasca do her work.

Do not go into this blindly. You must ask people who you know who have done this before to get direction on where to go for your ceremony. However, take their personal experiences with a grain of salt as everyone has a different experience with ayahuasca. Just because your friend had a certain kind of trip does not mean yours will mirror theirs even using the same retreat or shaman. It is up to the Spirit of the Vine to teach you what you need to know.

Since you likely are being drawn by Mother Ayahuasca to join in this experience, consider asking when you are deep in the ceremony to tell you why you were brought there. You might be surprised with what is presented to you.

Choosing the Best Shaman for You

Do not just show up to South America and expect for a Shaman to walk right up to you. In fact, if this happens, you need to head in the other direction. These again are charlatans who are taking advantage of the boost in ayahuasca tourism.

Cost of the retreats are not everything. There are centers that are a non-profit business and are just as reputable as high cost retreat centers. If you choose to go this route, look for your individual needs and how comfortable you feel about the place. Make sure to get all your questions answered and do not be embarrassed to ask anything. If they are reputable, the center will be transparent and honest in their answers with you.

Remember that the true healing Shamans are not going to be seeking praise or authority over you. They also are quiet and will not boast about their ability to heal you. Do not be pulled into this sham as it has already been discussed. Witch doctors only have ill intent in mind, and it is best to go in the other direction when confronted. Follow your intuition about a person who claims they have dealt with the Spirit of the Vine and dig deeper. Do not have any shame in asking them direct questions that you may even know the answers now after reading this book to see if they are being truthful.

Inquire about the specific ingredients in the brew. This is not a rude question as you only want to know what you are ingesting into your body. Also ask where it was made and by whom. This will also give you an idea of the authenticity of the process. If they have any admixtures that you are not knowledgeable about, do not partake until you have a full understanding of why these are being added and how that changes the traditional mixture.

Use your Intuition

If there is anything that rubs you the wrong way, this is your intuition going into high alert mode. If something does not feel or look right, investigate if you feel the need to do so or leave the retreat center if not in the middle of the ceremony except for extreme circumstances. Try to make friends if you are at a retreat center so that you can look after each other as much as you are able through the process. This will decrease the risk of inappropriate sexual encounters from happening or your partner being in distress and it going unnoticed by the facilitators and Shaman.

This is said for all genders as there have been reports of men, women and transsexuals being touched inappropriately. This is highly unlikely. However, you want to keep yourself protected as much as possible, especially when you are in a foreign land and incapacitated physically during the ceremony and psychologically afterwards.

When a Shaman uses their powers of manipulation and enchantment to take advantage of you in this vulnerable state, they are showing their true colors of being a sorcerer. You must break ties with his ceremonies and report these incidences with the local law enforcement and retreat center if you are attending one.

Sexual abstinence in the context of the spiritual realms brings you closer to the spirits as they reside at higher vibration levels, and it also brings clarity to your mind. This is seen in other spiritually based religions as a way to easily connect with your higher power.

Inner Work Homework

Do as inner work as possible before making the trip. If you do not practice a daily yoga or meditation session, start as soon as possible. This will align the energy in your body to your intention of your trip and will help the process go more smoothly than if you did not. If you are having major destructive behaviors that you are trying to break, seek counseling ahead of time to start peeling away at the root of the problem before cracking the whole issue at once in this sacred space. Have some personal responsibility and do not expect that Aya brew to cure your entire problem for you.

If your goal is to go through ego death, you must ponder upon the fact that you have lost the innocence you once had when you were younger. When you are born into this world, you are a clean slate and uncorrupted by your environment. You were curious and open to the ways of the world and had the capacity to love the world and the people within. If you look at your life now, you are likely trying to live by the standards of others and what they think of you, even if you try not to care. It in an adult's nature to compare themselves to their friends, coworkers or family and not be true to your authentic self. Judgement comes into the picture as your ego becomes developed with a sense of how we define ourselves to fit into the constructs of this world and thus you are bound by these ideas that society has set up. This is not an easy path to choose, but using ayahuasca to achieve this goal may be a fast track method to realize the obstacles that are in the way of you achieving this goal.

Honestly look at your attitude with the people you have long term relationship with as well as strangers you pass on the street. Do you need to adjust the way you approach these people so that these relationships can be elevated? Are there toxic people that need to be cut out of your entirely? This is your opportunity to gain insight and answers to these inquiries. Make the most of this experience.

It is important to ponder about root causes of emotional blockages as well as lacking qualities within close relationships you would like to address. If you are more in touch with your true personal state, this will help you to gain more awareness ahead of you drinking ayahuasca brew.

Because your thoughts have been on the subjects that you would like to aid in resolving, they will be more likely addressed during the ceremony. Also reflecting on the causes of your current state in all aspects of your life that need attention or cyclical occurrences of events in your life that seem to have no solution or perhaps you have a disconnect with the environment in which you live will also bring more awareness to these problems in your life.

It does not need to be a depressing assignment. As long as you are honest with yourself and where you stand, you will be more prepared to accept what is shown to you through Mother Ayahuasca so that you can finally break the cycles that are keeping you from rising and feeling an interconnectedness that gives your life meaning.

It is also helpful to talk to a friend or family member that you trust to be able to get a different perspective on your current state of affairs. Alternatively, a therapist who is certified in these matters would be able to give you some direction as well.

With this information in the forefront of your mind as well as going into the ceremony with no expectations, you will be able to surrender yourself more to the ceremony and flow with the energy that is presented. It will also give you the confidence that is required to see that whatever does transpire during the session is for your personal health and growth.

Trust & Respect

Before the ceremony or even arriving at the retreat center, you will likely sign an agreement or have a verbal understanding. This also needs to be respected like the Shaman and the medicine herself. Trust is absolutely necessary and broken agreements are a way to start off on the wrong foot. If you agreed to follow a certain regimen before arriving, you need to stick to it. If not, be honest with the parties involved to see if there is another measure to take or if you need to reschedule your ceremony.

Helpful Restrictions

Take care to keep your mental and physical state as clear as possible. Refuse any sexual encounters during the retreat, especially with the Shaman, and continue to refrain from sexual advances at least a week after the ceremony. The medicine may take longer than a week to work its way through your system. Use your judgement and extend the amount of self-care for as long as required during this integration period. If you feel pushed into any situation, kindly bow out and seek alone time to re-center.

Be Aware of Cultural Differences

Realize that the overall culture in South America is different, not just their religious belief system. The indigenous Amazonian men can have borderline chauvinistic attitudes towards women and do not recognize the same boundaries as they are understood in Western culture. This means that you may need to be less friendly than you are used to back home by not hugging or kissing someone on the cheek as you greet them or otherwise. This will be taken in a much different manner than just being kind and friendly.

This also means you need to be mindful about the clothes that you wear. You need to be respectful of the cultures of the people you will be surrounding yourself with as well as not give the wrong impression. You will find that you will be more welcome when you respect local dress code. This will also minimize unwanted curiosity and attention from the locals.

Get Comfortable

Follow the special dress code for the ceremony. Consider adding layers so that you can remove or put on clothes when your temperature fluctuates so that you are as comfortable as possible during the ceremony. If you have a certain crystal or spiritual items that you use in your personal worship, ask if it would be alright to bring them along as a comfort during this challenging journey or to simply charge them with the surrounding positive energies.

Integration Success

Do not forget the creative items to use to document your journey through drawings or insights you gained during the ceremony. This will keep the experience fresh in your mind as well as have them for visuals and notes later down the line. Perhaps you love to play a musical instrument. This is an excellent way to express your emotions in the days before and after the ceremonies to be able to channel your personal healing and perhaps of others.

While it is best for your purification and integration period to keep your subtle body energies at their peak, you must refrain from having any sexual or inappropriate relationships with your Shaman. If the Shaman is initiating this in any way, they are not a proper healer as they know this will only confuse the process further. Because you are under the influence of ayahuasca, you are not able to give any type of consensual interchange. This state of confusion can last for weeks after the ceremony itself and needs to be in the forefront of your aware mind.

The first week after your ayahuasca session is going to be the most intense. This is why it is stressed to start the integration period the day after the session. If the things you have experienced and realized during the ceremony are not recorded or expressed in some way, these encounters will be forgotten. With that said, do not make any rash decisions the day after the session either. Give yourself time to naturally come to these conclusions of what needs to alter drastically for at least 2 weeks if not longer after the event. If it is meant to happen, it will. There is no need to rush into things as it will help the process to just go with the current flow of things.

Coming Back to the Real World

You will find that you will not have the time or energy or care to dedicate to cultivating broken and toxic relationships. This automatically creates a space for healthy relationships based in compassion and love to flourish. When you come out of the mindset of being a victim to the deserved role of being the victor, your entire world is flipped on its ear in a good way, eventually.

As you can imagine, having all your beliefs shattered along with your perceptions altered, it can be an arduous task of picking up the pieces that are worth salvaging. This is where the integration period is an extremely important step. The session usually just takes place the day after the ceremony, but, in truth, it can last for months for a single ceremony. When you take the absolute truth of Mother Ayahuasca who you might have spoken with in her magical abode, it may seem difficult to compare the beautiful truth she presented to you and apply it in your life.

You will still need to go back to your old way of life and will have the same problems until they are dealt with head on. You will feel isolated from the event because you will not have anyone to relate to your experiences. You also will want to keep your personal revelations to yourself because they will only apply to you. So, in truth, people may ask you about your experiences, but you will not be able to express them or you will just want to keep it to yourself. You can use this time to be able to focus on the tasks that are at hand and do not get wrapped up in the same dramas that you were trying to heal in the first place when there are unwilling parties wanting the same result.

Your Health is Important

If you are on any medications or suffer from any physical and mental illnesses, you need to be upfront about this information with the facility or Shaman. It could mean the matter of life or death. There are healers that will work with people with certain ailments, so do not get discouraged if you want to try the avenue of ayahuasca as a second option

to what the medical doctors are prescribing. You have the right to seek alternative help, and the true Shamans will help you if they are able.
Even when you stop taking the medication in anticipation for your upcoming ceremony, keep your medication with you at all times. You never know if you may need it. Do not get discouraged if you should need to go back onto your medication for health reasons. It could be a sign that you are not ready to drink ayahuasca as Madre Ayahuasca will make herself available to you when the time is right. Also, be aware that many of these ceremonies in the jungle are long distances from hospitals and may have difficult roads to get there otherwise. It is best to take precautions in these situations.
There are several natural supplements and medications that are incompatible and even dangerous to combine with ayahuasca. The main culprits are anti-depressants, SSRIs and MAOI prescriptions. As mentioned, these can be detrimental to your health, causing mental and physical ailments, even including death. These need to be stopped at least one month prior to the ceremony. If they are required for your overall health, consult your medical doctor to discuss your options. Even following the recommendation of stopping these medications and supplements, you need to disclose your use of these items with the Shaman or retreat center so that they can be aware and inquire further if needed.
To add to the list are nicotine and recreational drugs as these will react adversely to the MAOI inhibitors in the Aya brew, even causing death. There are differing lengths recommended to avoid these items anywhere from 2 days to 3 weeks. Your facilitator or Shaman will inform you what they feel is best for you personally.
Sexual activity, including masturbating, is to be avoided for at least 2 weeks prior to drinking the brew. The sexual energy that is contained in your body through your kundalini is a powerful asset to keep at the highest levels during the ceremony. This will ensure you will experience the highest level of hallucinations, gaining the most insight from Madre Ayahuasca.
It is highly important to your health to make sure that certain medications and supplements are not present in your body during the ayahuasca ceremony. Your medical doctor needs to be involved in the process to ensure your health is guarded while you wean yourself off of your medication safely. Know that there are differing times that

medications and supplements fully leave the body so your preparation time for the ceremony may vary depending on which medication or combination of medications has been ingested over time.

Be sure to follow their recommendations and inform the Shaman or retreat center of any medications that you have been prescribed. This is a list of the most common negative impact prescriptions and supplements that will interact negatively with the ingredients and effects of the ayahuasca brew.

- Alcohol
- Anti-psychotics
- Central Nervous System (CNS) or anxiety depressants
- Anti-histamines
- Caffeine
- Nicotine
- Asthma or other breathing medications
- Diet pills
- High blood pressure medications
- Amphetamines
- Selective serotonin reuptake inhibitors (SSRIs)
- Sinicuichi
- Yohimbe
- Ginseng
- Ephedra
- Kava
- St. John's Wort
- Barbiturates
- Vasodilators
- Sleeping pills
- Migraine medications
- Mescaline
- Nasal sprays

Prepare for Travel

When you are traveling to the Amazon to receive the medicine, know that there is a great divide in social classes that you are going to encounter. Not everyone has good intentions and there is not always law enforcement readily available in case you should need them. When you are traveling, keep an eye on your luggage and have plans ahead of time for transportation to and from the airport in secured taxis or other form of transport. When you are in larger cities, it is best not to walk alone at night, and be diligent during the day because crimes can happen at any time.

South America has gotten a bad rap for being a dangerous place to visit, and it has much improved over the years as tourism has skyrocketed. These tips are given as a common sense measure. You would be diligent to your safety to any foreign country that you happen to visit.

If you are visiting the jungles of the Amazon, know that the humidity and heat can be overwhelming to someone who is not used to these conditions. This weather brings along with it insects, sweating and unpredictable monsoon like rains. On the other hand, in the mountains a person would likely encounter altitude sickness as well as the heat. Know that the temperatures drop drastically in the shade so it is best to stay out of the sun as much as possible.

Because of the possible extreme changes in climate and surroundings, it is best to schedule your arrival at least a few days before you are to partake in the ayahuasca tea ceremony. This will allow your body to rest from your travels as well as to adjust to your new surrounds to make the ceremony go smoother. This is also coupled with making sure your mind is in a calm state before the ceremony.

The main language in South America is Spanish. However, you will find in the more rural indigenous communities of the Amazon that they will speak their own languages such as Quechua. Plan ahead of time if you feel you will need a translator or make sure to have a good understanding of the Spanish language before venturing to South America.

CONCLUSION

I hope you enjoyed *Ayahuasca Awakening: The Truth Behind the Amazon Jungle's Sacred Plant Medicine.* Let us hope it gave you all of the information that you were searching for how to use this master plant to help you heal you in every way that you crave.

The next step is to follow the guidelines for finding a retreat center or shaman to work with and start planning your trip to South America or other location of your choice. Remember, it is not recommended to do this on your own, especially for your first experience.

Use the detailed list of preparation tips to ensure that you are as prepared as possible and open your heart and mind to the endless possibilities of what can happen.

I hope that this gave you the hope that there are magical ways that ayahuasca can heal your life physically, mentally and spiritually. I do wish you a fantastic encounter where you are able to realize your full potential.

Good luck in taking the step towards living your life in a more thoughtful and meaningful way.

Very grateful thanks for reading all the information included in your new book. Hopefully it has given you the wisdom and confidence that you need to take your first step in your Ayahuasca journey.

Finally, if you found this book useful in any way, a review on Amazon is always appreciated! Thank you!

DESCRIPTION

If you ever asked yourself who you really are on the inside and wanted to get down to the bottom of this question in a raw, honest and transparent way, ayahuasca is a powerful medicine that will take you through the journey of realizing the answer to your question – and then some.

Have you ever contemplated on the thought that there must be more to life than this? Are we much more than just this limited form that walks aimlessly on this earth? Do you want to be able to realize the immense energy that resides in you, yes YOU?

When you enter into the multiple level healing world of ayahuasca, you can connect with this infinite energy which will transform your health as well as your physical and spiritual wellbeing in a way you could never imagine.

If it is healing of a past traumatic event, disease that you have been battling, or you simply want to know your purpose in this life, this is the book that you need to get you the results that you are searching for.

Everything you need to know about what to expect during the ceremony as well as preparation and integration tips are included inside. This guide will give you the insight into the complete picture of the world of the healing medicine of Ayahuasca.

So get your copy of *Ayahuasca Awakening: The Truth Behind the Amazon Jungle's Sacred Plant Medicine* so you can learn how to change your life for the better starting today!

CPSIA information can be obtained
at www.ICGtesting.com
Printed in the USA
BVHW041637030621
608739BV00003B/842

9 781955 617444